Window to
Psoriasis

Window to
Psoriasis

Sharmila Patil

MD DDV (Mum.)

Professor and Head
Department of Dermatology
DY Patil University School of Medicine
Nerul, Navi Mumbai
Maharashtra, India

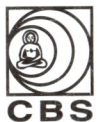

CBS Publishers & Distributors Pvt Ltd

New Delhi • Bengaluru • Chennai • Kochi • Kolkata • Mumbai
Hyderabad • Jharkhand • Nagpur • Patna • Pune • Uttarakhand

Window to
Psoriasis

ISBN: 978-93-85915-07-9

First Edition: 2016

Reprint: **2017**

Published by Satish Kumar Jain and Produced by Varun Jain for

CBS Publishers & Distributors Pvt Ltd

4819/XI Prahlad Street, 24 Ansari Road, Daryaganj, New Delhi 110 002, India.

Ph: 23289259, 23266861, 23266867   Website: www.cbspd.com

Fax: 011-23243014   e-mail: delhi@cbspd.com; cbspubs@airtelmail.in.

Corporate Office: 204 FIE, Industrial Area, Patparganj, Delhi 110 092

Ph: 4934 4934   Fax: 4934 4935   e-mail: publishing@cbspd.com; publicity@cbspd.com

Branches

- **Bengaluru:** Seema House 2975, 17th Cross, K.R. Road, Banasankari 2nd Stage, Bengaluru 560 070, Karnataka
  Ph: +91-80-26771678/79   Fax: +91-80-26771680   e-mail: bangalore@cbspd.com
- **Chennai:** 7, Subbaraya Street, Shenoy Nagar, Chennai 600 030, Tamil Nadu
  Ph: +91-44-42032115   Fax: +91-44-42032115   e-mail: chennai@cbspd.com
- **Kochi:** Ashana House, No. 39/1904, AM Thomas Road, Valanjambalam, Ernakulum 682 016, Kochi, Kerala
  Ph: +91-484-4059061-65   Fax: +91-484-4059065   e-mail: kochi@cbspd.com
- **Kolkata:** 6/B, Ground Floor, Rameswar Shaw Road, Kolkata 700 014, West Bengal
  Ph: +91-33-2289-1126, 1127, 1128,   e-mail: Kolkata@cbspd.com
- **Mumbai:** 83-C, Dr E Moses Road, Worli, Mumbai-400018, Maharashtra
  Ph: +91-22-24902340/41   Fax: +91-22-24902342   e-mail: mumbai@cbspd.com

Representatives

• **Hyderabad**	0-9885175004	• **Jharkhand**	0-9811541605	• **Nagpur**	0-9021734563
• **Patna**	0-9334159340	• **Pune**	0-9623451994	• **Uttarakhand**	0-9000660880

Printed at Magic International, Greater Noida, UP

Foreword

Psoriasis is a frequently encountered disease in clinical practice and presents itself in various clinical forms from just nail pitting to extensive body involvement in erythrodermic psoriasis, the management of which is often difficult. This book is intended to give practitioners, whether consultants, family physicians or medical students, a quick glance into the essential features of various presentations of psoriasis and guide the reader in their management.

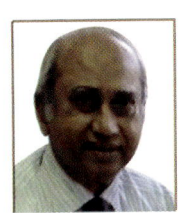

Clinicians will do well to get an essence of the problem from this book and then go to a more exhaustive work should they want to know more.

The book has many interesting features, beginning with an approach to a patient with psoriasis, its etiopathogenesis, to the management of erythrodermic, pediatric and nail psoriasis. It also discusses topical, systemic and phototherapy in psoriasis. The risk of tuberculosis with the use of TNA-α antagonists, a topic of importance to those intending to use biologics in India, is well discussed, so also the use of dermatoscopy in psoriasis.

This book has a wealth of information, written by teachers with a lot of experience, in a lucid style, that will no doubt be of a great benefit to the patient it is intended to manage.

Dr Rui Fernandes
MD, DVD, DDV
Professor Emeritus
Department of Dermatology
Seth GS Medical College and
KEM Hospital, Mumbai
Former President, IADVL

Contributors

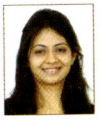

Aayushi Mehta
Resident
DY Patil University School of
Medicine
Nerul, Navi Mumbai
Maharashtra, India

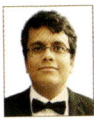

Aditya Mahajan
Resident
DY Patil University School of
Medicine
Nerul, Navi Mumbai
Maharashtra, India

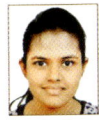

Amita Mhatre
Resident
DY Patil University School of
Medicine
Nerul, Navi Mumbai
Maharashtra, India

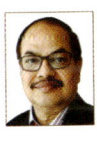

Arun C Inamadar
Professor and Head
Sri BM Patil Medical College
and Hospital
BLDE University, Bijapur
Karnataka, India

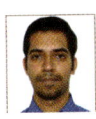

Harsh Tahiliani
Resident
DY Patil University School of
Medicine
Nerul, Navi Mumbai
Maharashtra, India

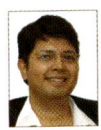

Kaleem Khan
Dr Nina Madnani's Skin Clinic
Colaba, Mumbai
Maharashtra, India

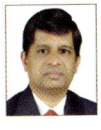

Kiran V Godse
Professor
DY Patil University School of
Medicine
Nerul, Navi Mumbai
Maharashtra, India

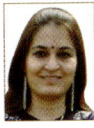

Manjyot M Gautam
Associate Professor
DY Patil University School of
Medicine
Nerul, Navi Mumbai
Maharashtra, India

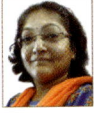

Meghana Phiske
Assistant Professor
LTMMC and LTMG Hospital
Sion, Mumbai, Maharashtra,
India

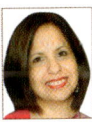

Nina Madnani
Visiting Consultant
PD Hinduja National Hospital
and Sir HN Reliance
Foundation Hospital
Mumbai, Maharashtra, India

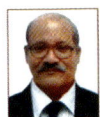

Nitin Nadkarni
Professor
DY Patil University School of
Medicine
Nerul, Navi Mumbai
Maharashtra, India

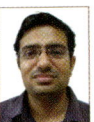

Parag Chaudhari
Assistant Professor
DY Patil University School of
Medicine
Nerul, Navi Mumbai
Maharashtra, India

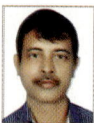
Parag Sharma
Associate Professor
Terna Medical College
Nerul, Navi Mumbai
Maharashtra, India

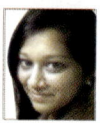
Pranjal Mittal
Resident
DY Patil University School of
Medicine
Nerul, Navi Mumbai
Maharashtra, India

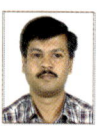
Ragunatha S
Professor
Sri Siddhartha Medical
College
Tumkur, Karnataka, India

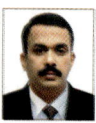
Sathish Pai B
Professor and Head
Kasturba Medical College
Manipal, Karnataka, India

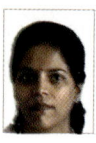
Sharmila Patil
Professor and Head
DY Patil University School of
Medicine
Nerul, Navi Mumbai
Maharashtra, India

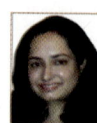
Shweta Agarwal
Assistant Professor
DY Patil University School of
Medicine
Nerul, Navi Mumbai
Maharashtra, India

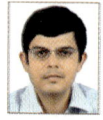
Sujay Khandpur
Professor
All India Institute of Medical
Sciences
New Delhi, India

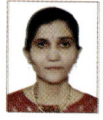
Sunanda Mahajan
Associate Professor
GS Medical College and
KEM Hospital
Mumbai, Maharashtra, India

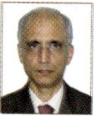
Sushil Tahiliani
Consultant Dermatologist
Asian Heart Institute
Hinduja Health Care
Mumbai, Maharashtra, India

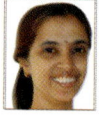
Vidya Kharkar
Professor
Seth GS Medical College
and KEM Hospital
Parel, Mumbai
Maharashtra, India

Preface

Psoriasis is one of the most common debilitating diseases seen in private practice. It is a disease with many interfaces including dermatology, rheumatology, immunology and (with the recent association of psoriasis with metabolic syndrome) in internal medicine too. Even a surgeon may encounter psoriatic lesions at the site of operation and may have to rapidly diagnose the case. The quality of life is affected depending on the extent of disease and the occupation of the person.

The morphological presentation also varies. This book is meant primarily for dermatologists, but also for general practitioners with an interest in dermatology, physicians, rheumatologists and internists. Hence this book aims to assist the consultants in their busy practice to diagnose, investigate and treat the patients optimally using newer drugs. The authors of each chapter have been chosen on the basis of their expertise in the field to provide the best guidance to our readers.

Sharmila Patil

Contents

Approach to a Case of Psoriasis

Nitin Nadkarni, Aayushi Mehta

"The fact that psoriasis is compatible with good physical health and that it is not easily treated must account, in part, for the neglect it has suffered."

—*John T Ingram, 1953*

Psoriasis is a chronic autoimmune condition, with a relapsing and remitting course. It can be controlled with various available medications, leading to symptomatic improvement; however, no known cure exists.

A patient of psoriasis will present to the OPD with one or more of the following symptoms:

1. Acute shower of guttate lesions.
2. Slowly progressing scaly plaques over certain sites of predilection.
3. Diffuse redness and scaling involving almost entire body, either occurring in the plaques aforementioned, or occurring *de novo*.
4. Localised or diffuse eruption of pustules usually occurring suddenly, either *de novo* or in a patient with pre-existing plaques.
5. Pain and stiffness in the joints, either the large weight bearing joints, spine, or small joints of fingers and toes.
6. Localised eruptions on scalp, flexures, genitals, palms and soles, and nail.
7. Deep fissures, thickening of the palms and soles.
8. Discoloration, thickening and cosmetic disfigurement of the nails.

HISTORY TAKING

A common approach can be formulated if a proper history and examination is done. The following points are important in the history:

1. *Presence of itching*: Though classical teaching is that psoriasis is non-itchy, it is not always so. The importance of itching is that it can trigger new lesions of psoriasis due to Koebner phenomenon.

2. *Duration*: Psoriasis is often a chronic relapsing disease with winter exacerbations.

3. *Initial site*: Classic psoriasis often begins on the scalp, in the gluteal cleft (Abrahamowitz sign), or at sites of injury and trauma. It may be mistaken for several years as a case of "dandruff", intertrigo or contact dermatitis.

4. *Mode of spread*: A rapid spread of psoriatic lesions is characteristic of type I psoriasis (young age, positive family history), while the opposite is true of type II psoriasis.

5. History of *pustule* formation or *pain* in the skin is observed in pustular or erythrodermic psoriasis.

6. In guttate psoriasis, there may be a history of previous sore throat; in pustular psoriasis, there may be a history of taking systemic drugs like steroids, anticonvulsants, or antimalarials; in erythrodermic psoriasis, there may be a history of exposure to antimalarials and anti-hypertensives. Table 1.1. lists drugs causing or exacerbating psoriasis.

7. *Systemic features*: In erythrodermic and pustular psoriasis, there would be history of fever, shivering, facial and lower limb puffiness or edema, palpitations and breathlessness.

Table 1.1: Drugs associated with onset or exacerbation of psoriasis

- Lithium, lithium salts
- Antimalarials (chloroquine, hydroxychloroquine)
- Beta-blockers
- NSAIDs
- ACE inhibitors
- Withdrawal of corticosteroids
- Gold salts
- Topical anthralin and coal tar (irritant effect)

8. In case of suspected joint psoriasis, the following 5 questions are useful to ask (*GRAPPA criteria*):[1]
   - History of pain or swelling in the joint
   - Whether any doctor has told the patient that he was suffering from arthritis
   - Pain in the heel
   - Nail involvement
   - History of painful or swollen finger or toe without injury

9. *History of treatment taken:* A detailed history of treatment taken in the recent as well as remote past, especially alternative medicine treatments, since they often contain minerals like mercury and arsenic which may be toxic to the patient. Also ask whether the treatment has improved or worsened the psoriasis.

10. *History suggestive of systemic complications of psoriasis:* Psoriasis is often associated with metabolic syndrome (diabetes, obesity, hypertension, hyperlipidemia) and symptoms of bowel disease.

11. *Personal history:* History of promiscuous sexual activity (HIV is known to precipitate or exacerbate psoriasis, and lesions of secondary syphilis and Reiter's disease can mimic psoriasis). History of recent weight loss (early mycosis fungoides can mimic psoriasis and HIV can also trigger psoriasis). History of alcoholism, known to worsen psoriasis, especially of facial distribution. History of smoking—known to worsen palmoplantar pustular psoriasis.

12. *Family history:* First degree or second degree relatives suffering from similar lesions or arthritis, or bowel disease, increases the probability of the patient having psoriasis.

13. *Quality of life:* History of disability, limitations in daily activities, interpersonal relations affected, effect on job and economic situation of the family. History of stress precipitating the disease, worsening the disease, or being caused due to the disease.

CLINICAL EXAMINATION[2]

Some diagnostic guidelines have been proposed in literature on the basis of clinical features.[3] Presence of all the following features together greatly improves the specificity of diagnosis:

1. Characteristic morphology of erythema, scaling, and induration
2. Scalp involvement
3. Nail involvement
4. Involvement of the intertriginous folds
5. Family history of psoriasis

Chronic Plaque Psoriasis

The classical **MADE** approach should be followed:

M   Morphology: The lesions are scaly plaques of various sizes and shapes, some of which may show central clearing, and also may show circinate borders. Always elicit Auspitz sign, candle wax sign, both of which are positive in psoriasis and also elicit deep dermal tenderness (Buschke-Ollendorff sign which will be negative in psoriasis). Look for the Woronoff ring (halo of hypopigmentation), which indicates healing psoriasis.

A   Arrangement: The lesions are mostly symmetrical. Often the lesions are linear (Koebner's phenomenon) or annular or geographic.

D   Distribution: The extensors, classically—elbows, knees, lumbosacral region, palms, soles, scalp, nail are usually involved.

E   Evolution: The lesions start as small papules, evolve into larger plaques, may heal in the centre, may spread peripherally, occasionally show small pustules and heal with hypo-pigmentation but no scarring.

Guttate Psoriasis

M   The lesions are small, erythematous, drop-like macules and papules. Auspitz sign is usually negative, and the lesions are non-scaly.

A   The lesions are symmetrical and koebnerisation is negative.

D   Usually on the trunk.

E   Starts as macules and evolves into papules.

Erythrodermic Psoriasis

M   Patient has diffuse erythema and scaling all over the body, sometimes, occasional scaling plaques are seen at the borders of the erythema. The scales are usually thin, and on removal, can leave behind diffuse bleeding rather than pinpoint. The skin is often thickened, but lichenification is usually absent.

A Lesions are symmetrical.

D Lesions are generalized. Very often flexures, and tip of the nose (Pavithran's sign) are spared.

E The lesions start as small papules and rapidly spread to give diffuse erythema, scaling and thickening (exfoliative dermatitits).

Pustular Psoriasis

M The lesions are small follicular and non-follicular pustules, but, can enlarge to form 'lakes' of pus on erythematous skin. The lesions are tender. Nikolsky's sign is negative.

E The patient initially has diffuse erythema, followed by pustules which enlarge to form large lakes of pus which dry up and exfoliate. Lesions in different stages of evolution are present in the same patient.

Arthropathic Psoriasis

Look at the fingers, and palpate joints for swelling, tenderness, and crepitus. Test the mobility of important joints like knees, ankles, fingers, hip by putting the joint through the proper range of movement. Palpate the spine and tap the sacroiliac joint. Feel for warmth over any swollen joint.

Nail Psoriasis

Look for the 8 signs of nail involvement:

Nail matrix involvement: (1) Pitting, (2) Crumbling, (3) Red lunula, (4) Leuconychia.

Nail bed involvement: (1) Subungual hyperkeratosis, (2) Onycholysis, (3) Salmon patch/oil drop sign, (4) Splinter hemorrhages.

Total number of pits in both fingers and toes should be more than 20 to be significant. Look at palms and soles for plaques or pustules.

Scalp Psoriasis

Look at the scalp for diffuse scaling, circumscribed plaques, or lesions in the rim of the scalp (corona psoriatica).

Genitals

In uncircumcised patients, there may be only erythema and maceration without scaling. In circumcised patients, there will be regular erythematous scaly papules. On the labia, there may be erythematous, scaly papules and plaques, which may be lichenified.

Mouth

There may be chronic migratory glossitis on the tongue.

Eyes

Look at the eyes to rule out Reiter's disease.

DIFFERENTIAL DIAGNOSIS

Differentials of chronic plaque psoriasis:
1. Secondary syphilis
2. Reiter's syndrome
3. Parapsoriasis
4. Atopic dermatitis
5. Seborrheic dermatitis
6. Psoriasiform eczema
7. Pityriasis rubra pilaris
8. Discoid lupus erythematosus

Differentials of scalp psoriasis:
1. Seborrheic dermatitis
2. Pityriasis sicca
3. Tinea capitis
4. Secondary syphilis—corona veneris
   (Four causes of corona on the scalp—corona syphilitica/veneris, corona seborrheica, corona psoriatica, corona of Reiter's disease)

Differentials of palmoplantar psoriasis:
1. Psoriasiform eczema
2. Hypertrophic lichen planus
3. Secondary syphilis
4. Palmoplantar keratodermas
5. Porokeratosis of Mibelli
6. Palmoplantar pustulosis (some people consider it a variant of psoriasis)

Differentials of guttate psoriasis:
1. Guttate pityriasis rosea
2. Guttate parapsoriasis

3. Pityriasis lichenoides chronica
4. Lichen planus

Differentials of flexural psoriasis:
1. Tinea cruris
2. Candidiasis
3. Hailey-Hailey disease
4. Bowen's disease
5. Paget's disease

HISTOPATHOLOGY

Although biopsy is not routinely required for diagnosis of psoriasis, it is very useful in doubtful and atypical cases to rule out differentials such as psoriasiform eczema.

Chronic Plaque Psoriasis

- Parakeratosis of stratum corneum
- Loss of granular layer
- Neutrophils in stratum corneum (Munro's microabscesses)
- Regular acanthosis
- Thickening of rete ridges in lower portion (clubbing)
- Thinning of suprapapillary epidermis
- Capillary dilatation and edema in papillary dermis
- Extravasation of WBCs, mainly lymphocytes from dilated blood vessels
- Rarely, neutrophilic *spongiform pustule of Kogoj*, with adjacent mild spongiosis
- *Sandwich sign*—collection of neutrophils alternating with parakeratosis in the startum corneum

Pustular Psoriasis

- *Spongiform pustule of Kogoj*, often as macropustule (aggregation of neutrophils in upper spinous layer)
- Formation of large pustules in epidermis in generalized pustular psoriasis
- Large Munro's abscesses
- Parakeratosis
- Elongation of rete ridges.

Guttate Psoriasis

- A focus of neutrophils above an area of parakeratosis (*half sandwich sign*).

DERMOSCOPY

Dermoscopy is becoming a very important investigation in confirming the diagnosis of psoriasis. It has the advantage of being non-invasive and helps to rule out differentials. Dermoscopy in psoriasis should always be performed after removal of scales for visibility. In chronic plaque psoriasis, multiple red globules in a honeycomb or sieve-like pattern. For further details, refer to the chapter on dermoscopy in psoriasis.

Investigations

Table 1.2: Investigations in a case of psoriasis

Investigations to confirm the diagnosis:
- Skin biopsy
- Dermoscopy
- HLA B 27 testing in case of psoriatic arthropathy
- Throat swabs and ASO titres in guttate psoriasis
- Pus smear and culture in pustular psoriasis

Investigations to rule out differential diagnosis:
- VDRL
- Skin biopsy (eczema, lichen planus)
- KOH mount (dermatophytosis)
- HIV

Investigations for associations and complications:
- Serum lipid profile
- CBC
- FBS, PLBS
- BP and cardiac monitoring when indicated
- LFT
- HBsAg

ASSESSMENT OF SEVERITY OF PSORIASIS

There are a multitude of tools which have been described in literature to assess the severity of psoriasis, nail psoriasis, and psoriatic arthropathy, along with their various modifications. However, we will focus on the more popular tools which are useful in a day-to-day clinical practice.

Psoriasis Area and Severity Index (PASI)

The PASI score is currently the most utilized tool in assessment of psoriasis, especially in various trials evaluating the efficacy of treatments for psoriasis. It was first described in 1978[4] and has since then been widely published and modified as per clinical requirements.

PASI score can be calculated as follows:[4]

	Head	Upper limbs	Trunk	Lower limbs
Redness (0 to 4)	$R_H =$	$R_U =$	$R_T =$	$R_L =$
Induration (0 to 4)	$I_H =$	$I_U =$	$I_T =$	$I_L =$
Scaling (0 to 4)	$S_H =$	$S_U =$	$S_T =$	$S_L =$
Total	$T_H = R_H+I_H+S_H$	$T_U = R_U+I_U+S_U$	$T_T = R_T+I_T+S_T$	$T_L = R_L+I_L+S_L$
Area Score[#] (0 to 6)	A_H	A_U	A_T	A_L
Area multiplier	0.1	0.2	0.3	0.4
PASI	$(0.1 \times T_H \times A_H) + (0.2 \times T_U \times A_U) + (0.3 \times T_T \times A_T) + (0.4 \times T_L \times A_L)$			

[#]Area Score: 0: 0 (clear) 1: < 10% 4: 50–< 70%
2: 10–< 30% 5: 70–< 90%
3: 30–< 50% 6: 90–< 100%

The final PASI score can vary between 0.0 and 72.0. PASI 75 response is a ≥75% reduction from the baseline PASI score. This is the benchmark endpoint used in most clinical trials for assessment of psoriasis therapies.[5] However, some authors have considered this too stringent, and even a PASI 50 response has been described in literature as being clinically meaningful.[5]

Disadvantages of PASI[5,6]

- Upper end of the scale is only theoretical
- Weak responsiveness when patients reach < 10%BSA (changes with lesser body surface areas do not easily reflect in PASI)
- Considerable experience required for good reliability
- Time and resource intensive tool
- Complex
- Lacks sensitivity
- Non-linear scale

Modifications of PASI Score[6]

1. *Self-administered PASI (SAPASI)[7]:* A structured PASI—like instrument designed for patient's self-assessment of severity. Patient's shade areas of body affected in a line drawing and grade severity of erythema, induration, scaling by visual analog scales. The investigator calculates the SAPASI score. This score has been found to correlate well with PASI score, also showing good responsiveness to changes in severity with treatment.

SAPASI score	Clinical severity of psoriasis
SAPASI = 0	In remission
0 < SAPASI < 3	Mild
3 < SAPASI < 15	Moderate
SAPASI > 15	Severe

2. *Simplified PASI:* The simplified PASI equals the sum of the average redness, thickness, and scaling of all the psoriasis lesions, multiplied by an estimate of total percentage body surface area involved. It is meant to be easy to use. However, adequate studies on reliability are lacking and it seems to be less sensitive to change.

3. *Modified PASI for palmoplantar psoriasis:[8]* Head and trunk have to be taken as 0. Upper limbs modified as palms, lower limbs as soles. The areas of involvement are scored accordingly.

Physician Global Assessment (PGA)[8]

The Physician's Global Assessment is typically a 7-point scale. It can be either dynamic PGA or static PGA, depending on whether a comparison is made with baseline scores. However, the dynamic one would require recall or baseline photographs, and hence is less frequently used. It has the disadvantage of not reflecting small changes easily.

Score	Rating	Description
7	Severe	Very marked plaque elevation, scaling, and/or erythema
6	Moderate to severe	Marked plaque elevation, scaling, and/or erythema
5	Moderate	Moderate plaque elevation, scaling, and/or erythema

Contd...

Score	Rating	Description
4	Mild to moderate	Intermediate between moderate and mild
3	Mild	Slight plaque elevation, scaling, and/or erythema
2	Almost clear	Intermediate between mild and clear
1	Clear	No signs of psoriasis (postinflammatory hyperpigmentation may be present)

The score can be interpreted as 0 = Clear, 1–5 = Increasing severity, and 6 = Worsened.

Some other scoring systems in psoriasis are
1. Psoriasis severity scale
2. Salford psoriasis index
3. Nail psoriasis severity index
4. Psoriasis assessment severity score (PASS)
5. Lattice system physician's global assessment (LS-PGA)
6. Psoriasis disability index
7. The National Psoriasis Foundation—Psoriasis Score (NPF-PS).

However, description of each of these is beyond the scope of this book and the reader is directed to refer the material cited below for further information.

FINAL DIAGNOSIS

It should include:
1. Type I or Type II psoriasis
2. Morphological type of psoriasis
3. Activity of psoriasis
4. Area of involvement
5. PASI score
6. Presence or absence of nail or joint involvement
7. Presence or absence of metabolic syndrome

REFERENCES

1. Ibrahim GH, Buch MH, Lawson C, Waxman R, Helliwell PS. Evaluation of an existing screening tool for psoriatic arthritis in people with psoriasis and development of a new instrument: the PEST questionnaire. Clin Exp Rheumatol 2009;27(3):469–74.

2. Wielowieyska-Szybinska D, Wojas-Pelc A. Psoriasis: course of disease and treatment. Post Dermatol Alergol 2012;XXIX,2:118–22.
3. Johnson MA, Armstrong AW. Clinical and histologic diagnostic guidelines for psoriasis: a critical review. Clin Rev Allergy Immunol 2013;44(2):166–72.
4. Fredriksson T, Pettersson U. Severe psoriasis-oral therapy with a new retinoid. Dermatologica 1978;157:238–44.
5. Feldman SR, Krueger GG. Psoriasis assessment tools in clinical trials. Ann Rheum Dis 2005;64(Suppl II):ii65–8.
6. Spuls PI, Lecluse LL, Poulsen ML, Bos JD, Stern RS, Nijsten T. How good are clinical severity and outcome measures for psoriasis?: quantitative evaluation in a systematic review. J Invest Dermatol 2010;130(4):933–43.
7. Fleischer AB Jr, Rapp SR, Reboussin DM, Vanarthos JC, Feldman SR. Patient measurement of psoriasis disease severity with a structured instrument. J Invest Dermatol 1994;102(6):967–9.
8. Specific Disease Scores. In: Krupashankar DS, Sacchidanand S(Eds) Scoring Systems in Dermatology, 1st ed. New Delhi: Jaypee Brothers Medical Publishers; 2009, p. 50–61.

2

Epidemiology and Etiopathogenesis of Psoriasis

Sharmila Patil, Amita Mhatre

INTRODUCTION

Psoriasis is a chronic inflammatory and hyperproliferative skin disorder with increasing prevalence. It is a chronically relapsing disease with high morbidity and impaired quality of life. It is characterized by erythematous scaly plaques affecting skin, joints, and nails. Psoriasis is identified as a marker of metabolic syndrome with multiple co-morbid associations like cardiovascular diseases and diabetes mellitus. Psoriasis is a disorder of immune system. Genetic, immunologic and environmental factors are implicated in the etiopathogenesis of psoriasis. Understanding of psoriasis at the molecular level has improved the management of psoriasis. Newer specifically targeted biologics and immunosuppressive agents have made achievement of long-term remission possible.

HISTORY

The term 'psora' was first used by Galen. Robert Willan in 1809 gave an accurate description of psoriasis and Hebra in 1841 distinguished features of psoriasis from leprosy. In case of treatment, exposure to sunlight was the oldest treatment.

EPIDEMIOLOGY

Psoriasis is found worldwide with vast differences in the prevalence among different parts of the world due to genetic and environmental factors that greatly influence the clinical development of the disease. Population based studies have revealed prevalence ranging from 0.2% to 4.8%. The highest prevalence rate from recent population surveys is seen in Denmark and Norway, with reported prevalence of 7.1% and 8.5%.[1] The incidence of psoriasis appears to be lower in Asians with recorded prevalence of about 0.3%.[2] Psoriasis is known to affect 1–2% of the population in the US.

Age: Psoriasis may first appear at any age from birth to old age, although more likely to occur between 15 and 30 years of age. Henseler and Christopher showed that certain HLA class I antigens, particularly HLA-Cw6 is associated with early age of onset and with a positive family history. Depending on this, there are two clinical presentations of psoriasis: type I disease with age of onset before 40 years, positive family history, HLA associated with refractory and severe course; and type II psoriasis without HLA association or family history.[3]

Sex: Psoriasis is equally common in males and females. Indian studies report slight preponderance in males.

GENETICS OF PSORIASIS

The role of genetics in psoriasis is well recognized. The inheritance is multifactorial, requiring polygenic and environmental factors for its clinical expression. The most susceptibility factor for psoriasis is Cw6 allele in the PSORS1 region.[4] It is associated with type I disease and exacerbation following streptococcal infection. There are many other MHC class I and II molecules associated with psoriasis. HLA-B27 is associated with psoriatic arthritis.

Other reported psoriasis susceptibility loci are:

- PSORS2 locus situated near the telomeric end of chromosome 17q.
- PSORS3 locus on chromosome 4q34 associated with early-onset psoriasis with a gene coding for a protein that regulates the production of type 1 interferon.[5]
- PSORS4 locus resides within the epidermal differentiation gene complex on chromosome 1q21.
- PSORS5 locus on chromosome 3q21.
- PSORS6 locus on chromosome 19p13 that harbors the JUNB gene that controls keratinocyte differentiation.[6]

Recently, PSORS9 is reported that harbors gene that codes for immunologically relevant proteins, including interleukin 15 gene.[7]

IMMUNOPATHOGENESIS

Psoriasis is T cell dependent autoimmune disease. The concept of immunological component to the pathogenesis of psoriasis was made by serendipitous observation that patients receiving an immunosuppressive drug, who also had psoriasis, found that their disease was clearing.

Psoriasis is a hyperproliferative disorder with inflammation and altered differentiation. The proliferation is mediated by complex cascade of inflammatory mediators.

The milieu of psoriatic skin immunologically includes T lymphocytes CD4+, CD8+, neutrophils, mast cells, macrophages and dendritic cells. Specific steps must occur in sequence to result in T cell activation.

Immune activation occurs through antigen presenting cells (dendritic cells) processing antigen, migrating to regional lymph nodes and stimulating the naïve cells to become active Th1 and Th17 cells that return to skin via expression of CLA (cutaneous leukocyte antigen) and LFA-1, IFN, TNF. There is expression predominantly of cytokines like IL-2, INF-α, TNF-α. Further, they induce keratinocytes to produce adhesion molecules such as ICAM-1, costimulatory molecules like CD 40 and MHC II molecules, VGEF, IL-8. Recently described cytokines, apart from IL-6, IL-8, that are expressed in psoriatic lesions include IL-15, IL-19 and IL-20 that influences keratinocyte proliferation.[8]

The disease initiation is suggested to be mediated through dendritic cells (DC's) presenting foreign antigen or self-antigens to T-lymphocytes. HSP70 expressed by keratinocytes and HSP70 receptor CD91 by dermal DC's may result in autostimulation.[9]

Following are a few triggering factors:

- Infections (streptococcal via superantigen activation)
- Psychogenic stress
- Drugs (commonly hydroxychloroquine, lithium, NSAIDs, carbamazapine, β-blockers) (Table 2.1)
- Alcohol
- Smoking
- Obesity
- Endocrine (hypocalcemia has been known to precipitate pustular psoriasis).

Table 2.1: Drugs that trigger psoriasis

Association	Class
Known	β-blockers Lithium Hydroxy-/chloroquine
Likely	Tetracycline ACE inhibitors Non-steroidal anti-inflammatory drugs (NSAIDs) Interferons Terbinafine
Case reports	Multiple
"New"	Efalizumab and transient neutrophilic dermatosis TNF-α blockers and pustular transformation of plaque-type psoriasis

Leptin is found to induce keratinocytes to secrete pro-inflammatory cytokines, thus increasing the severity of psoriasis in patients with high body mass index.[10]

Keratinocyte Growth and Differentiation

The balance between keratinocyte production in the basal layer and corneocyte shedding at the skin surface is required for maintaining equilibrium of the normal epidermis. This balance is affected in psoriasis due to altered keratinocyte growth and differentiation.

The proteins like keratins, involucrin, psoriasin, fatty-acid binding protein, calgranulins A and B, cystatin show altered expression in psoriatic skin as compared with normal skin.[11]

The transcription factor STAT-3 is expressed by the lesional epidermal keratinocytes which may upregulate ICAM-1 and TGF-α, which is known to stimulate proliferation in psoriasis.

These sequences of events manifests as hyperproliferative epidermis, lymphocyte infiltration mostly of T lymphocytes, various endothelial vascular changes in dermis, such as angiogenesis, dilatation and endothelial venule formation. The epidermal mass is increased 3–4 times the normal skin. The granular cells are vacuolated focally and disappear, with parakeratosis seen above this area. Neutrophils that are periodically discharged from

Steps in Pathogenesis of Psoriasis

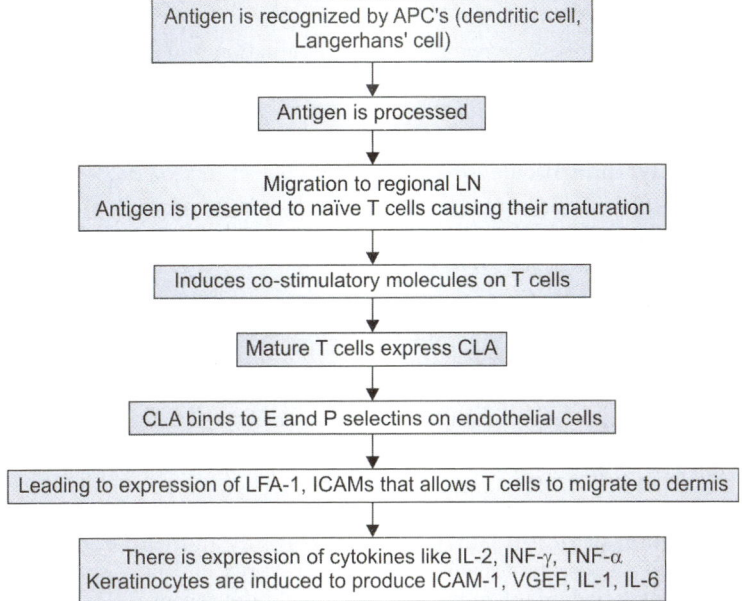

the capillaries, are attracted to parakeratotic areas forming Munro's microabscess. Sometimes neutrophils may aggregate in spinous layer resulting in 'spongiform pustule of kogoj'.

The same is clinically evidenced as erythematous, dry, scaly plaques with silvery scales. The extent of involvement of skin can range from discrete localized lesions to generalized involvement of the body.

With the better understanding of etiopathogenesis of psoriasis, the newer molecules can be identified as targets for biological therapy which promises long-term remission

REFERENCES

1. Bo K, Thoresen M, Dalgard F. Smokers report more psoriasis, but not atopic dermatitis or hand eczema: results from a Norwegian population survey among adults. Dermatology 2008;216:40–5.
2. Yip SY. The prevalence of psoriasis in the Mongoloid race. J Am Acad Dermatol 2001;26:314–20.
3. Henseler T, Christophers E. Psoriasis of early and late onset: characterization of two types of psoriasis vulgaris. J Am Acad Dermatol 1985;13:450–6.

4. Nair RN, Stuart PE, Nistor I, et al. Sequence and haplotype analysis supports HLA-C as the psoriasis susceptibility 1 gene. Am J Hum Genet 2006;78:827–51.

5. Forester J, Nolte I, Schweiger S, et al. Evaluation of the IRF-2 gene as a candidate for PSORS3. J Invest Dermatol 2004;122:61–4.

6. Lee YA, Ruschendorf F, Windemuth C, et al. Genome-wide scan in German families reveals evidence for a novel psoriasis-susceptibility locus on chromosome 19p13. Am J Hum Genet 2000;67:1020–4.

7. Willasden LS, Schurman J, Beurskens F, et al. Resolution of psoriasis upon blockade of IL-15 biologic activity in a xenograft mouse model. J Clin Invest 2003;112:1571–80.

8. Rückert R, Asadullah K, Seifert M, et al. Inhibition of keratinocyte apoptosis by IL-15: a new parameter in the pathogenesis of psoriasis? J Immunol 2000;165:2240–50.

9. Boyman O, Conrad C, Dudli C, Kielhorn E, Nickoloff BJ, Nestle FO. Activation of dendritic antigen-presenting cells expressing common heat shock protein receptor CD91 during induction of psoriasis. Br J Dermatol 2005;152:1211–8.

10. Xue K, Liu H, Jian Q, Liu B, Zhu D, Zhang M, Gao L. Leptin induces secretion of pro-inflammatory cytokines by human keratinocytes *in vitro*—a possible reason for increased severity of psoriasis in patients with high body mass index. Experimental dermatology 2013;22:406–10.

11. Mckay IA, Leigh IM. Altered keratinocyte growth and differentiation in psoriasis. Clinics in dermatology 1995;13:105–14.

3

Types of Psoriasis

Shweta Agarwal

The diagnosis of psoriasis is mainly clinical since the most common presentation is chronic plaque psoriasis characterised by plaques with silvery white scales and Auspitz sign positivity. However, the other variants of psoriasis may cause some diagnostic difficulties. It is imperative to know the types or the classification of psoriasis to diagnose correctly, for treatment purpose and to predict the course and outcome.

Psoriasis may be Classified on the Basis of

a. *Age of onset*
Type I psoriasis—age of onset before 40 years
Type II psoriasis—age of onset after 40 years

b. *Degree of severity (BSA)*
<5% BSA—mild
5–10% BSA—moderate
>10% BSA—severe
Localised/widespread psoriasis

c. *Pattern of distribution*
Inverse, seborrheic

d. *Morphology*
Plaque, guttate, erythrodermic, pustular, rupoid, elephantine

e. *Site*
Scalp, palmoplantar, genital, nail

f. *Disease activity*
Stable/unstable

1. *Psoriasis vulgaris (chronic stationary psoriasis, plaque-type psoriasis)*
(Figs 3.1 to 3.3)
It is the most common type of psoriasis seen in 90% of the
patients. The lesions are erythematous with silvery white
scales, symmetrically distributed plaques localized to the

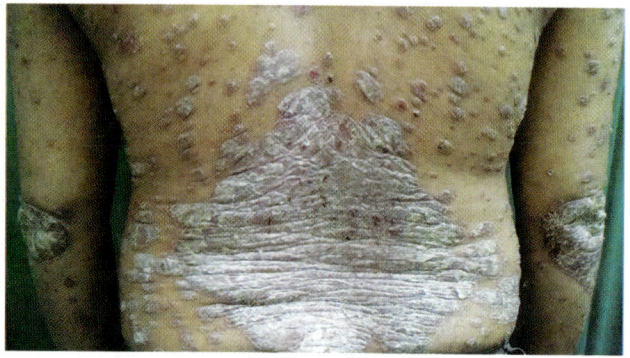

Fig. 3.1 Chronic plaque psoriasis

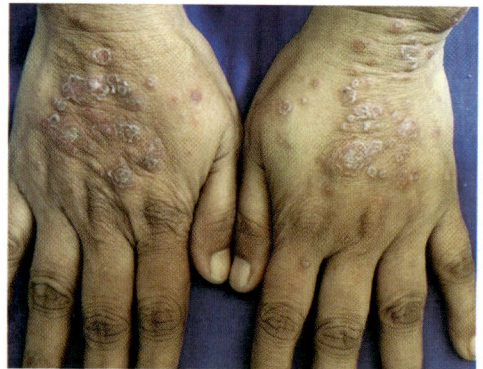

Fig. 3.2 Chronic plaque psoriasis

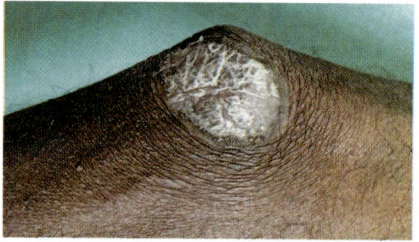

Fig. 3.3 Chronic plaque psoriasis

extensor aspects of extremities along with scalp, lower lumbo-sacral region, buttocks and genital involvement.

Other sites: Umbilical, intergluteal cleft.

Variants:

1. *Psoriasis geographica*
   The smaller lesions coalesce to form plaques whose borders resemble a map.
2. *Psoriasis gyrate*
   The lesions extend laterally and become circinate.
3. *Annular psoriasis* (Figs 3.4 and 3.5)
   The lesions show partial central clearing which results in ring-like lesions. This variant has good prognosis.

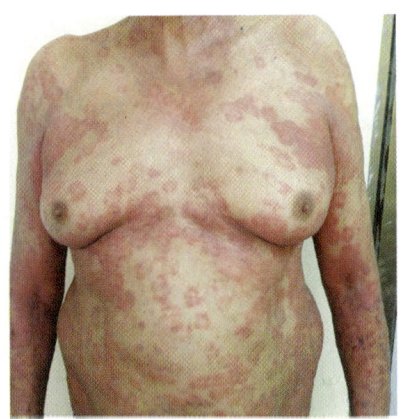

Fig. 3.4 Annular plaque psoriasis

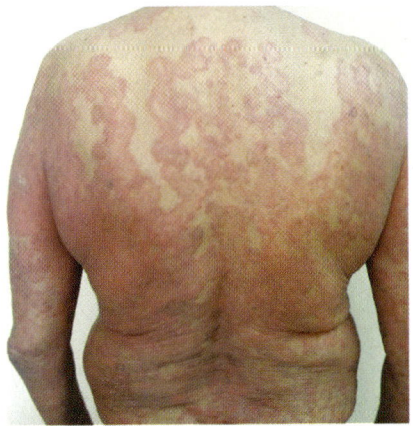

Fig. 3.5 Annular plaque psoriasis

4. *Rupoid psoriasis*
   The lesions are shaped as a cone or limpet.

5. *Ostraceous psoriasis*
   Lesions are hyperkeratotic concave lesions resembling oyster shell.

6. *Elephantine psoriasis*
   It is an uncommon variant. Lesions are thick scaly large plaques usually on lower extremities.

2. *Guttate (eruptive) psoriasis* (Figs 3.6 and 3.7)
   Derived from Latin word 'gutta' meaning a drop.

   Incidence: 1.9% of the psoriasis affected population

   The body shows eruption of small (0.5–1.5 cm) papules over the trunk and proximal extremities. It typically manifests at an early age, frequently found in young adults.

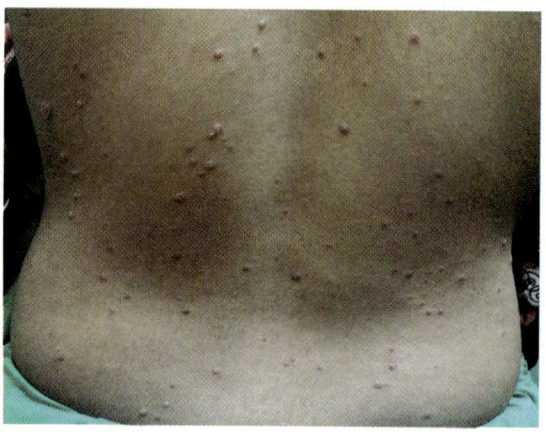

Fig. 3.6 Guttate psoriasis

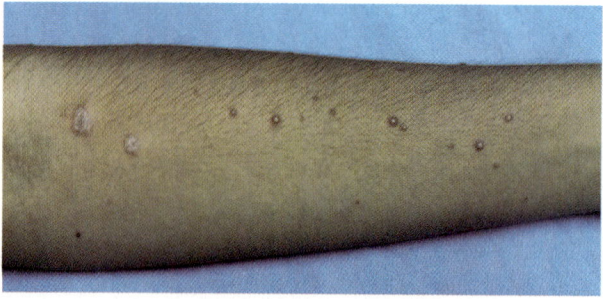

Fig. 3.7 Guttate psoriasis

This form has the strongest association with HLA-Cw6. Streptococcal throat infection frequently precedes onset or flare of guttate psoriasis.

It can also be seen in patients with chronic plaque psoriasis.

3. *Small plaque psoriasis*

It is common in Korea and other Asian countries. The lesions resemble guttate psoriasis and occur in older individuals. The lesions are slightly larger, thicker and scalier than guttate lesions.

4. *Palmo-plantar psoriasis* (Figs 3.8 to 3.10)

Psoriasis presents as typical scaly plaques with fine silvery scales which may be elicited by grattage. The lesions may resemble lichen simplex or eczema. Sharply demarcated

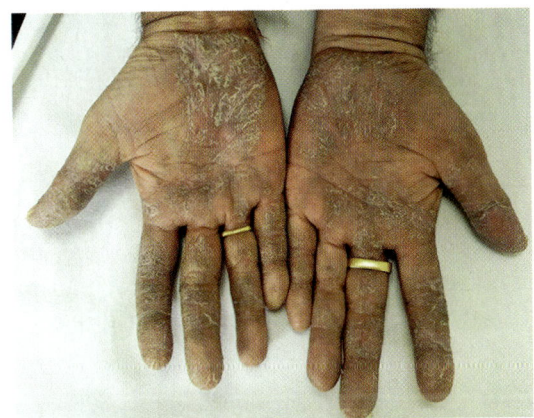

Fig. 3.8 Palmar psoriasis

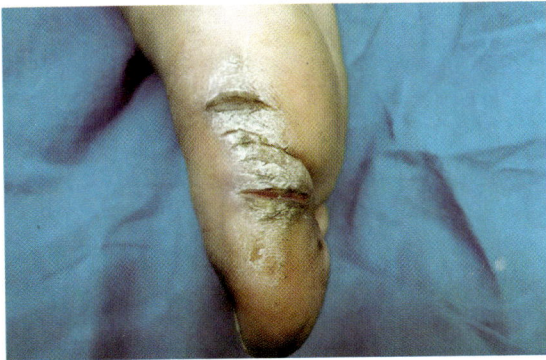

Fig. 3.9 Localised plantar psoriasis with fissures

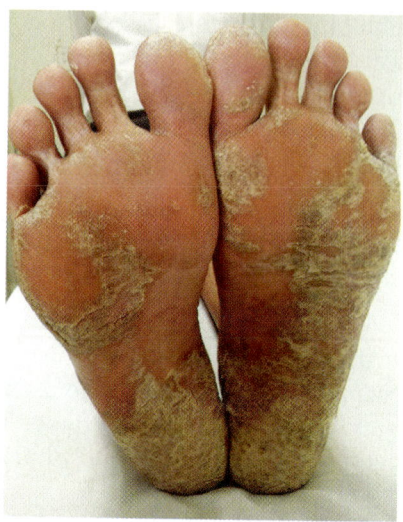

Fig. 3.10 Plantar psoriasis

borders of the lesions help to distinguish it from eczema. It may be precipitated by occupational irritants.

5. *Inverse (flexural) psoriasis* (Fig. 3.11)

   Incidence: It is more common in older individuals than children.

   It may occur as a primary disease or Koebner phenomenon on top of infective or seborrhoeic intertriginous dermatoses.

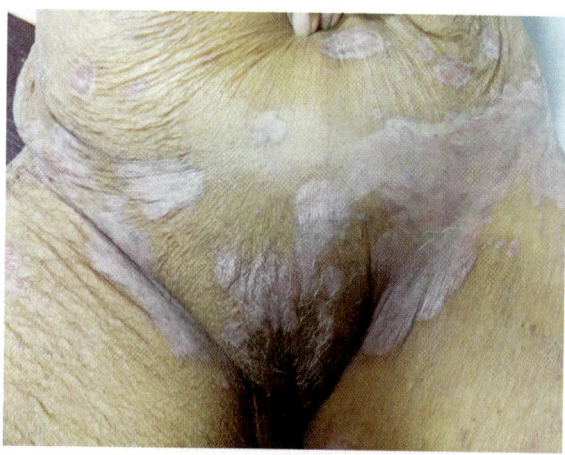

Fig. 3.11 Inverse psoriasis

It is seen in the axillae, genito-crural region and the neck. Scaling is minimal or absent, surface is glossy with sharply demarcated erythema and may show fissuring in the centre of the fold. The lesions are anhidrotic and the surrounding area may show hyperhydrosis.

6. *Erythrodermic psoriasis* (Fig. 3.12)

   Incidence: 1–2.25%.

   It affects more than 90% of the body surface area. Erythema is the most prominent feature. The scaling is superficial. Loss of heat occurring due to generalized vasodilatation causes hypothermia.

   Psoriatic skin is hypohidrotic due to occlusion of sweat ducts leading to a risk of hyperthermia in warm climates. Lower extremity edema, high-output cardiac failure, impaired renal function may occur.

   Chronic form:

   Plaque psoriasis worsens to involve entire body and patients respond better to treatment.

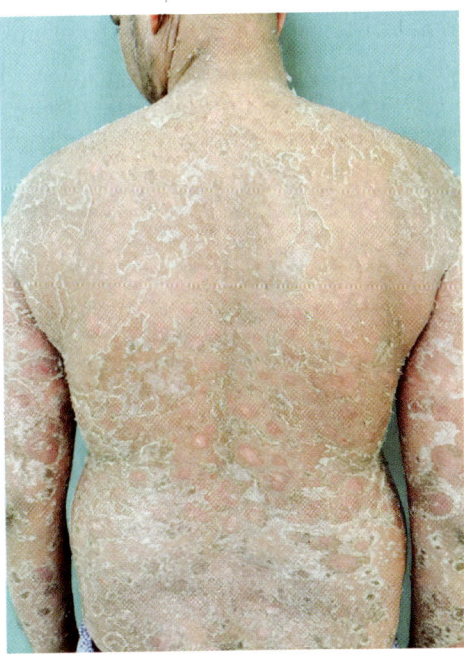

Fig. 3.12 Erythrodermic psoriasis

Acute form:

Sudden generalised erythroderma as a result of intolerance to therapy representing a generalised Koebnerisation.

7. *Pustular psoriasis*

   Variants: (a) Generalised pustular psoriasis (von Zumbusch type): (i) Impetigo herpetiformis, (ii) Annular pustular psoriasis. (b) Localised pustular psoriasis: (i) Pustulosis palmaris et plantaris, (ii) Acrodermatosis continua of Hallopeau.

   a. Generalised pustular psoriasis. It presents as sudden generalised eruption of sterile pustules 2–3 mm in diameter over trunk and extremities with fever for several days. The nail bed, palms and soles are also involved. Pustules arise in highly erythematous skin and become atrophic. The disease occurs in waves of fever and pustules.

   Provoking agents are infections, irritation by topical treatment and withdrawal of oral steroids. This type of psoriasis is associated with systemic symptoms and life-threatening complication.

   Drugs used commonly for treatment are etretinate, methotrexate, cyclosporine, infliximab or oral steroids.

   b. Exanthematic pustular psoriasis (Fig. 3.13): This type tends to occur after a viral infection. It does not show constitutional symptoms and does not tend to recur. There can be a overlap

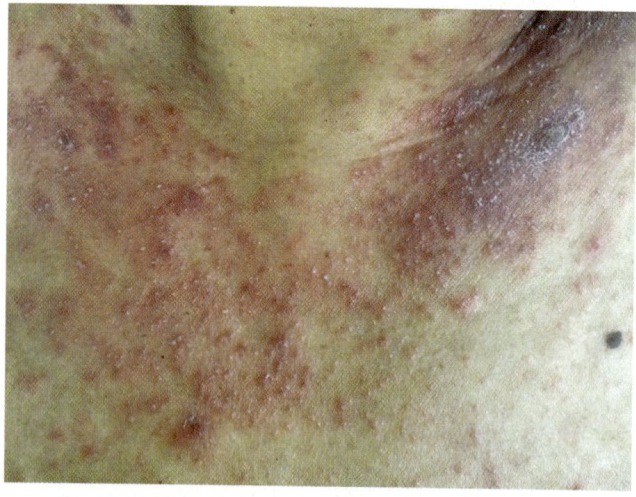

Fig. 3.13 Exanthematic form of pustular psoriasis

between this and acute generalised exanthematous pustulosis.

c. Annular pustular psoriasis: It is a rare variant of pustular psoriasis. It presents as annular or circinate form at the onset of pustular psoriasis or may develop during the course of generalised pustular psoriasis. It can occur in the early 3rd trimester of pregnancy and persist until delivery. It is often associated with hypocalcemia. There is no personal or family history of psoriasis.

d. Localised pustular psoriasis (Fig. 3.14): Palmoplantar pustulosis: This is located to palms and soles. More common in females, seen in 5th–7th decade and associated with smoking. These are well-defined erythematous scaly plaques with numerous tiny yellow pustules distributed bilaterally, symmetrical on thenar and hypothenar eminences of the palms, soles and side of the heels.

Acrodermatitis continua of Hallopeau: This is believed to be a variant of LPP. There is chronic, pustular lesions starting at the tip of digits that extend locally. Subtle trauma generally preceeds the lesion that start as glazed erythema of fingertip covered by scales. Subsequently, minor pustules appear with involvement of nail and digits become painful.

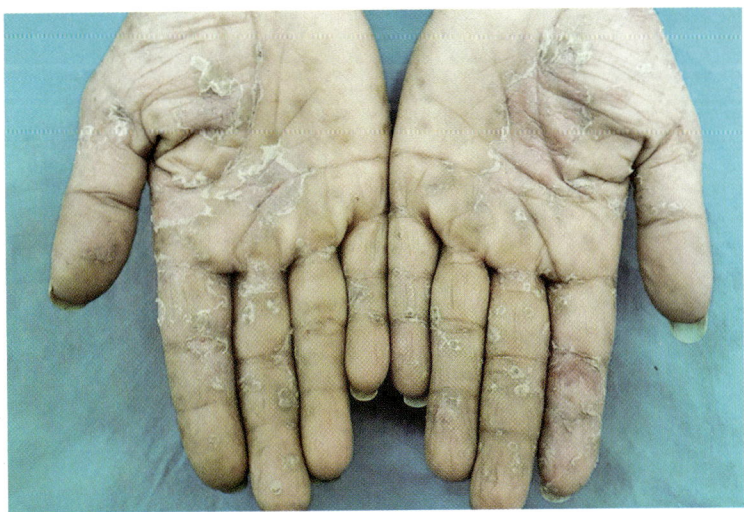

Fig. 3.14 Healing pustular psoriasis

8. *Linear psoriasis*

It is a very rare form. The typical psoriasis lesions appear on limbs and sometimes on trunk along a dermatome. It is regarded as a form of ILVEN.

9. *Unstable psoriasis*

It denotes the phases of psoriasis in which the disease activity is marked and the course of disease and the immediate outcome is unpredictable. It may be precipitated by withdrawal of intensive systemic or topical corticosteroid therapy, hypoglycemia, acute infection, overtreatment with tar preparations, phototherapy or stress.

10. *Scalp psoriasis* (Fig. 3.15)

Around 50–80% patients have either scalp psoriasis alone or along with lesions elsewhere. Scalp psoriasis is found mostly in children and adolescents. The patient usually complains of scaling or redness on the scalp with occasional itching. It may present as well-defined erythematous plaques with silvery scales or a diffuse involvement which may be difficult to distinguish from seborrheic dermatitis. The scales in seborrheic dermatitis are greasy and lesions rarely extend beyond the hairline, whereas in psoriasis, the scales are dry and lesions

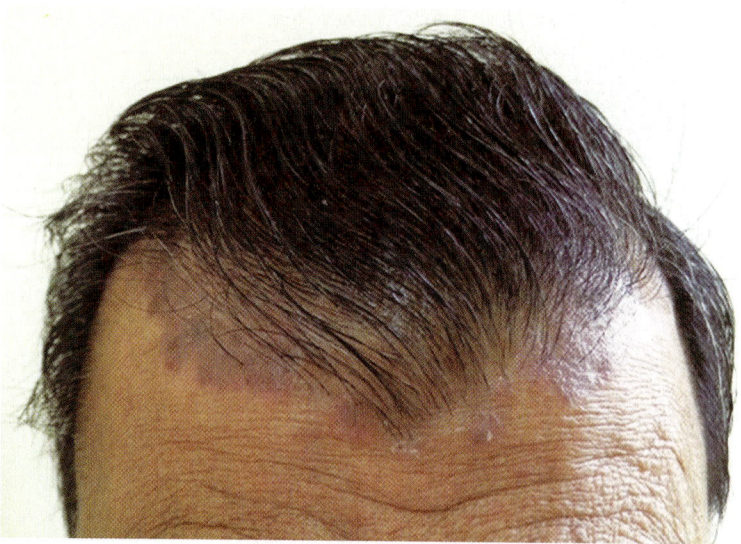

Fig. 3.15 Scalp psoriasis

extend beyond the hairline. The other variants seen are pityriasis amiantacea and sebopsoriasis. Psoriasis Disability Index and Scalpdex are two tools which can be used to determine the quality of life of the patient.

Pityriasis (tinea) amiantacea

It is a non-specific reaction pattern common in children and young adults. It is characterised by thick plaques with asbestos-like scaling firmly adherent to the scalp and hair. There may be cicatricial alopecia.

Sebopsoriasis

It is characterised by erythematous plaques with greasy scales localised to seborrheic areas. It may represent a modification of seborrheic dermatitis on a genetic background of psoriasis. It is relatively resistant to treatment.

11. *Nail psoriasis* (Figs 3.16 and 3.17)

    Classical nail involvement is useful in confirming the diagnosis of psoriasis in doubtful cases. Pitting of nails is the most characteristic feature, whereas onycholysis is the most common nail abnormality in psoriasis. Involvement of the nail bed is often represented by the appearance of orange-yellow areas beneath the nail plate known as "oil spots". Subungual hyper-keratosis is seen in chronic cases. Nail Psoriasis Severity Index (NAPSI), modified NAPSI, target NAPSI, Psoriasis Nail Severity Score, Nail Area Severity are various scoring systems used to measure the severity of psoriasis.

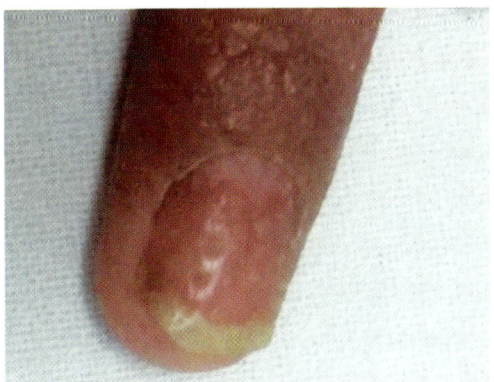

Fig. 3.16 Nail psoriasis

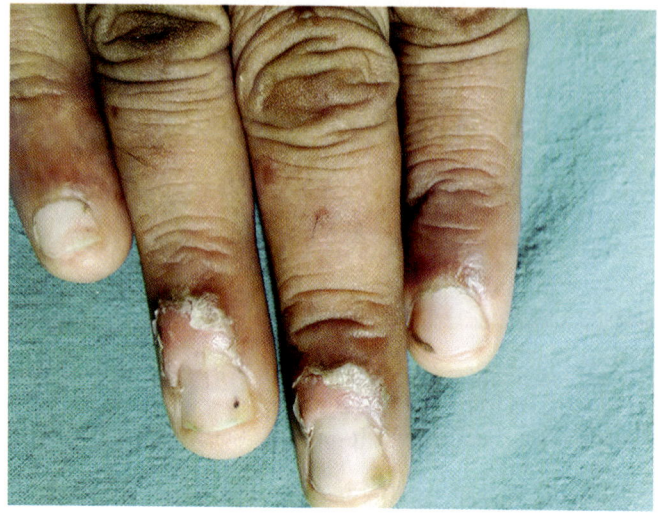

Fig. 3.17 Nail psoriasis

12. *Napkin psoriasis* (Fig. 3.18)

It begins at 3–6 months and presents as confluent red area with appearance of small red papules the napkin area and appear on the trunk and limbs a few days later. The face may also be involved. It responds well to treatment and disappears at the age of one year.

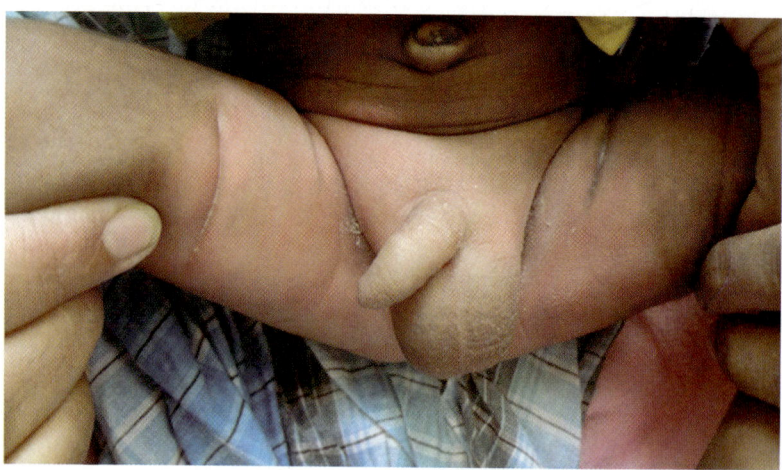

Fig. 3.18 Napkin psoriasis

Childhood Psoriasis

Approximately one-third of the patients develop psoriasis in the first two decades of life. Congenital psoriasis is rare. Localised psoriasis especially face, guttate psoriasis and napkin psoriasis are common in children. 38% having facial involvement and 26% having napkin psoriasis were found in an Australian study of childhood psoriasis.

Ocular Psoriasis

Conjunctivitis, blepharitis, keratitis, xerosis, trichiasis, chronic uveitis and symblepharon may be seen.

RECOMMENDED READING

1. CEM Griffiths, JNWN Baker. Psoriasis. In: Tony Burns, Stephen Breathnach, Neil Cox, Christopher Griffiths (Eds). Rook's Textbook of Dermatology, 8th edn, Vol. 1. Wiley-Blackwell, 2010;20:1–60.

2. Morris A, Rogers M, Fischer G, Williams K. Childhood psoriasis: a clinical review of 1262 cases. Pediatr Dermatol 2001;18:188–98.

3. SK Raychaudhari et al. Autoimmunity reviews 2014;13:490–95.

4

Erythrodermic Psoriasis

Meghana Phiske

INTRODUCTION

Erythroderma, a rare and severe cutaneous syndrome, is characterized by presence of a confluent erythema and desquamation affecting more than 90% of the body surface with a prolonged course. Its annual incidence varies from country to country with 1–2 cases/100,000 inhabitants/year in Europe and USA.[1]

EPIDEMIOLOGY

Erythrodermic psoriasis (EP) is a rare subtype of psoriasis characterized by generalized erythema and scaling.[2] The estimated prevalence among psoriatic patients ranging from 1 to 2.25 % (frequency varies from 8.8% to 44.9%). Psoriatic origin seems most common in South Asia, Latin America and the Maghreb, especially in Tunisia (33% to 51.25% of erythrodermas).[1]

EP is more common in men during adulthood (mean age of onset ranging from 41 to 55 years), although it has been described in all ages, including rare congenital instances.[3]

Left untreated, it may lead to serious morbidity and even mortality,[4] with mortality rates of 15% and 9% (with 5% and 2% mortality rates attributable to psoriasis) even though the patients had received conventional treatments.[2]

ETIOPATHOGENESIS

Precipitating Factors

EP can result from aggravation of a previous case of unstable chronic plaque-type psoriasis or can appear as the initial presentation of psoriasis.[2]

Various precipitating factors include infection, drugs, over-treatment with tar or dithranol (representing a generalized Koebner's phenomenon), sudden withdrawal of potent topical or oral corticosteroids, cyclosporine, efalizumab or methotrexate, environmental, psychological and metabolic factors.[5-7]

Rebound after efalizumab discontinuation has been reported in patients with unsatisfactory clinical response. It may be due to down-regulation of cellular receptors and/or development of tachyphylaxis, defined as a rapidly decreasing response to a physiologically active agent after administration of a few doses.[3]

Phototherapy complications, severe emotional stress, and preceding illness are other precipating factors.[8] Widespread flares follow irritant contact dermatitis (e.g. tar) or systemic infection (HIV infection).[6]

The anti-TNF-α agents have rarely reported to trigger EP. The mechanism speculated being that TNF inhibition would lead to increased production of IFN-α by plasma-cytoid dendritic cells and local expression of type I IFN-induced genes in the skin of pre-disposed individuals, including chemokines CXCL9 and CXCL10, and overexpression of C-X-C motif receptor 3 and Tia-1 (involved in skin homing and cytotoxic activity, respectively) in T cells.[3]

EP triggered by intravesical bacillus Calmette-Guérin immuno-therapy,[9] Bupropion treatment to assist with cessation of smoking[10] and radiologic contrast media have been reported.[11] Recurrent erythrodermic psoriasis in a thiuram-allergic patient due to contact with nurses' rubber gloves has been described.[12] Table 4.1 gives the various triggering factors for EP.

Table 4.1: Various triggering factors for EP

Common	Uncommon
Infection	Bacillus Calmette-Guérin
Drugs	immunotherapy
Sudden withdrawal of potent topical	Bupropion treatment
steroids/oral corticosteroids, cyclosporine,	Radiologic contrast media
efalizumab or methotrexate	Rubber gloves
Overtreatment with tar or dithranol	
Environmental factors	
Psychological factors (severe emotional stress)	
Metabolic factors	
Preceding illness	
Phototherapy	

Role of Th Lymphocytes[3]

Although both T helper (Th)-1 and -2 lymphocytes are involved in the pathogenesis, EP patients exert a Th1/Th2 bidirectional response pattern, the balance of Th cell subsets inclines to Th2 causing Th1/Th2 imbalance with a relatively weak expression of Th1 and greater Th2 advantage. A similar assumption could justify the high level of immunoglobulin E (IgE) found in some EP patients.

The importance of Th2 response in EP is supported by the following evidence:

1. Th1/Th2 ratio in peripheral blood is significantly lower in EP patients than in those affected by psoriasis vulgaris.
2. Higher serum levels of interleukin (IL)-4 and -10, two important Th2 cytokines, are seen in EP as compared to psoriasis patients and a healthy control group.
3. Inverted ratios (1.0) of both interferon (IFN)-c/IL-4 (serum levels) and T-bet/GATA-3 (levels in both skin lesions and peripheral blood mononuclear cells) seen in EP patients.

Other Proposed Mechanisms[3,13]

1. A remarkable increase of Th1 cytokines such as IL-2 and IFN-c might be responsible for the development of EP, while a shift towards type 2 cytokine predominance would contribute to its resolution.
2. Interaction between lymphocyte adhesion molecules and their ligands. Increased concentration of circulating levels of soluble adhesion molecules (intercellular adhesion molecule 1, vascular cell adhesion molecule 1, and E-selectin) have been reported in EP patients compared with controls.

Classification[3]

EP may also be classified in two clinical subtypes.

1. *First form*:
   a. In this form chronic plaques gradually evolve into a generalized erythrodermic phase
   b. The psoriatic characteristics are retained (typical psoriatic plaques are seen)
   c. The disease is generally stable
   d. The prognosis is good.

2. *Second form*:
   a. It is part of spectrum of "unstable psoriasis"
   b. It is more common in arthropathic psoriasis
   c. It may occur any time presenting suddenly and unexpectedly or may appear after a period of increasing tolerance to local applications, UV therapy or loss of control over the disease.
   d. The characteristics of the disease are often lost (typically, an extensive erythema is observed, with or without scaling and no recognizable psoriatic plaque)
   e. Itching is often severe
   f. The disease is generally unstable
   g. Relapses are frequent
   h. The course is prolonged
   i. The patient may be febrile and ill
   j. There is a considerable mortality

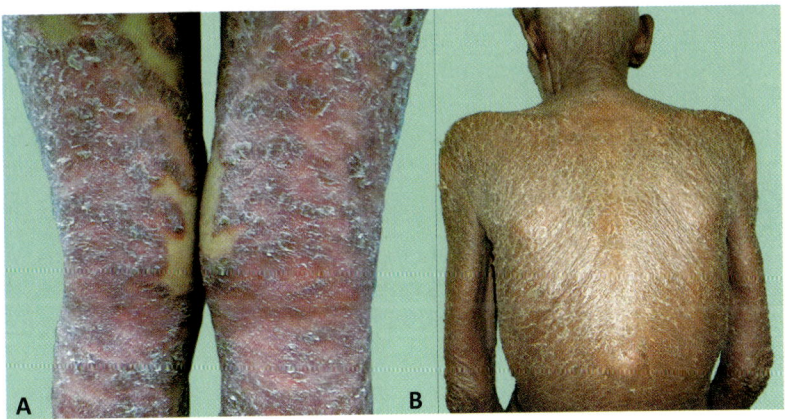

Fig. 4.1A and B Erythrodermic psoriasis (A) Type I and (B) Type II

Clinical Features

EP generally occurs in patients who already have chronic plaque-type psoriasis, but it may appear *de novo* onset in some patients. The average time interval between the onset of psoriasis and the first erythrodermic episode ranges from 11 to 18 years (3 weeks–42 years).[3]

   EP is the result of gradual progression of chronic plaque psoriasis with the plaques becoming confluent and extensive. It is characterized by diffuse red-violet erythema and fine scaling involving almost all of the body surface area. After generalization of the erythema, the typical features of psoriatic plaques are lost and disseminated sterile subcorneal pustules may develop.[6] Generalized pustular psoriasis may revert to erythroderma with diminished formation of pustules.[7] Treatment of the erythroderma may result in the reappearance of more characteristic psoriatic plaques.[6]

Skin scaling present is different from chronic plaque-type psoriasis as there is a superficial exfoliation rather than thick, adherent, white scales.[3] EP patients exhibit the "nose sign" which is near complete absence of erythema and scaling of the nasal and perinasal skin (to some extent), the reason for which is unknown.[7] Due to a slower turnover rate, nail changes, like oil-drop changes, onycholysis, onychodystrophy or nail pits may be visible providing valuable clue for diagnosis of EP.[6]

The erythematous-desquamative changes may be accompanied by weight loss, exudation, itch, widespread/lower extremity edema, mucosal involvement, hair loss, palmoplantar keratoderma, psoriatic nail changes and arthritis. The systemic manifestations include fever, chills, lymphadenopathy, malaise and fatigue.[3]

Erythrodermic verrucous psoriasis has been reported which can be diagnostic and therapeutic challenge.[14]

Complications of EP[3,7]

1. *Hypoalbuminemia*: It is due to high protein loss from scales.
2. *Lower limb edema*: It occurs due to hypoalbuminemia, increased capillary permeability and increased central venous pressure.
3. *Temperature changes*: Active inflammation causes increased blood flow through the skin and consequently excess heat loss from the body by convection and radiation. This compromises the temperature maintaning function of the body. The body tries to counteract the heat loss by shivering and by raising the basal metabolic rate which causes hyperpyrexia.
4. *Decreased sweating*: This results due to intraepidermal occlusion of eccrine sweat duct.
5. *Effects on cardiac output*: The increased cutaneous blood flow results in increased cardiac output and subsequently high cardiac output failure. The features of high output state include:
   a. Tachycardia
   b. High volume collapsing pulse

    c. Capillary pulsations

    d. Elevated jugular venous pressure

    e. High pulse pressure

    f. Cardiomegaly

    g. Apical systolic murmur

6. *Dermatogenic enteropathy*: This may cause malabsorption and secondary deficiency.

7. *Anemia*: Loss of large quantities of epidermal scales which are rich in proteins, iron, vitamin B_{12} and folate, cause deficiencies leading to anemia.

8. *Hypocalcemia*: It is consequence of hypoalbuminemia.

9. *Increased percutaneous absorption of topical preparations*: The impaired barrier function leads to increased percutaneous absorption of topical preparations, hence these should be used with caution.

10. *Oliguria*: Decreased renal blood flow leads to the risk of oliguria.

11. Shock and acute renal failure due to skin fluid loss.

12. *Lipomelanotic reticulosis*: This is referred to as generalized but benign enlargement of lymphnodes.

13. Sepsis from skin pathogens (especially *Staphylococcus aureus*).

14. Acute respiratory distress syndrome.

15. Hydroelectrolytic abnormalities.

Diagnosis

The evaluation includes:

1. *Detailed medical history*: Up to 45% of the patients will have a prior history of a more localized skin disease.[6]

2. *Clinical examination*: Accurate clinical examination may reveal additional clues to the underlying disease.[6] Final diagnosis can be made after excluding other differential diagnosis like drugs reactions, atopic dermatitis, infections, and malignancies (lymphoma and mycosis fungoides), which can be clinically indistinguishable from EP.[5]

3. *Histopathology*: Histopathological studies are also needed to arrive at a definitive diagnosis.[5] Although subtle, histopathologic features of the underlying disease are present in about two-thirds of patients. In 60% of EP patients, changes associated with

'early' psoriasis are found which include slight epidermal hyperplasia, a reduced or absent granular layer, focal parakeratosis, an edematous papillary dermis, and a perivascular, interstitial lymphohistiocytic infiltrate and occasional extravasated erythrocytes.[3] When features of early lesions of psoriasis are found during the evaluation of a biopsy specimen from a patient with a clinically nonspecific erythroderma, the diagnosis of psoriasis should be made.[14]

In 30% of patients with EP, histopathological findings are those of a fully developed psoriatic plaque and include epidermal hyperplasia with bottleneck-like rete ridges, confluent parakeratosis, absence of the granular layer, elongated dermal papillae, and a sparse lymphohistiocytic infiltrate.[3]

Ten percent of patients with psoriatic erythroderma exhibit findings of regressing psoriasis (i.e. slight epidermal hyperplasia, a normal or even thickened granular layer, and a fibrotic papillary dermis).[6] At times histologic examination is often non-specific, because the erythroderma modifies the usual histological signs of psoriasis, particularly frequent eczematization may cause epidermal spongiosis and lymphocytic exocytosis.[1]

Clues to the diagnosis of EP include previous plaques in classic locations, characteristic nail changes, and facial sparing. Table 4.2 gives the clues of EP.[6]

Table 4.2: Clues of psoriatic erythroderma

Clinical clues	Histologic clues	Additional hints
Presence of pre-existing psoriatic plaques	Confluent parakeratosis	Personal or family history of psoriasis
Sparing of the face	Bottleneck-like rete ridges	Withdrawal of corticosteroids or methotrexate
Presence of nail changes like oil-drop, pits, onycholysis	Tortuous vessels in papillary dermis	
Subcorneal pustules	Neutrophils in epidermis	
Inflammatory arthritis	Reduced granular layer	

Course of EP

The course of EP may vary from prolonged and chronic (more common for the first clinical subtype) to acute and rapidly progressive (more typical of the second clinical subtypes); sometimes, EP may follow a relapsing-remitting pattern, with classic plaques of psoriasis during remitting phases.[3]

Treatment

The management of EP is difficult and has not been standardized, posing a challenge to physicians, as currently available therapies often provide unsatisfactory results.[2]

Traditional systemic therapies effective for treating EP include:[2]
1. Methotrexate
2. Cyclosporine
3. Oral retinoid

Factors limiting use of traditional systemic therapies:[2,3]
1. Organ-specific toxicity
2. Inconvenience/intolerance
3. Risk of opportunistic infections
4. Treatment failure
5. Limited favorable outcomes (mortality rate of 9%)

Rationale for giving Anti-TNF-α Agent in EP[2]

In EP skin inflammation is the predominant feature and rapid systemic release of TNF-α may be responsible for the disease onset and severity. TNF-α is overexpressed in psoriatic skin lesions and promotes the proinflammatory cytokine cascade, leading to the recruitment of leukocytes to the lesional epidermis. Also TNF-α is distributed throughout the epidermis of lesional psoriatic skin and localized to the upper dermal blood vessels. Hence TNF-α is important in inducing and maintaining skin inflammation during psoriasis, which forms the rationale for using anti-TNF-α agent.

Recently Used Biological Therapies for EP[2]

1. TNF-α inhibitors
   Etanercept
   Infliximab
   Adalimumab
2. Anti-interleukin-12/23 p40 monoclonal antibody
   Ustekinumab

Advantages of Targeted Biological Therapies[2]

1. High selectivity for targeting specific pathways involved in the inflammation cascade
2. Have improved the safety profiles of several inflammatory arthropathies and psoriasis.

Drugs Recommended[3]

The 2010 (most recent) recommendations for the treatment of EP given by National Psoriasis Foundation Medical Board of the USA are:

First line therapy

- Acitretin
- Cyclosporine
- Methotrexate
- Infliximab

Second line therapy

- Etanercept and combination therapy
- Ustekinumab

Drugs not Recommended[3]

Systemic corticosteroids and UV light are not advised due to the possible flare upon withdrawal and significant photosensitivity of EP patients, respectively.

ACITRETIN[3]

Acitretin is generally used in EP with a low starting dose (25 mg/day), which is gradually increased until optimal response is achieved. A low starting dose helps to minimize the possible initial worsening of erythroderma related to the administration of relatively high doses of acitretin. First significant clinical effects are seen in about 4 weeks.

Combination with Acitretin

1. Infliximab and acitretin: Has been found effective.
2. Acitretin and cyclosporine: Failed to control EP in three patients in a case series.

CYCLOSPORINE[3]

Cyclosporine is the first line therapy for severe unstable cases of EP because of its rapid onset of action. The recommended starting dose is 5 mg/kg/day (slowly tapered after remission) cyclosporine can work in psoriasis induced by biological agents due to its peculiar suppressive activity on T lymphocytes and the concomitant specific action on keratocytes and angiogenesis.[15]

Combination with Cyclosporine

- Alefacept (one case)

- Methotrexate (two cases)
- Etretinate (six cases) (effective especially in patients not responding to monotherapy regimen).[16]
- All the above combinations have been reported to be effective.

METHOTREXATE[3]

Methotrexate is a valid and well-tolerated therapeutic option for EP, given in doses ranging from 7.5 to 40 mg/weekly. The first significant clinical results are generally seen within 1–4 weeks (faster than acitretin but slower than cyclosporine).

Miscellaneous Drugs

Other treatment modalities include mycophenolate mofetil,[17] short-course class 1 topical glucocorticoid under occlusion[18] and PUVA therapy and methotrexate.[19]

Complete resolution of EP in an HIV patient (unresponsive to antipsoriatic treatments) after highly active antiretroviral therapy has been reported.[20]

Summary of Drugs to be Used for EP

Table 4.3 gives the summary of drugs to be used for EP in adults.

Table 4.3: Summary of drugs to be used for EP in adults

Drug	Recommendation	Remarks
Acitretin	1st line	—
Cyclosporin	1st line	Rapid onset of action Preferred in acute, severe, unstable cases
Methotrexate	1st line	Rapid onset of action (faster than acitretin slower than cyclosporine) Well tolerated
Infliximab	1st line	Preferred in acute, severe, unstable cases Most frequently used Excellent response Rapid clearing (solo or combination)
Etanercept	2nd line	Useful in resistant cases
Ustekinumab	2nd line	Useful for long-term control Useful in resistant cases

ERYTHRODERMIC PSORIASIS IN PEDIATRICS

Epidemiology

Erythroderma is uncommon in children with an incidence of 0.11%. Psoriasis affects 0.12% to 0.71% of the population under 18 and psoriatic erythroderma accounts for 1.4% of psoriasis among children and adolescents.[21] In children psoriasis represents the second most common cause of erythroderma, after drug eruptions.[6] Cases of congenital or neonatal EP are rarer.[22]

Etiopathogenesis

Trauma, infections, drugs, environmental, psychological, and metabolic factors are the triggering factors. Poor specificity of clinical and histological features leads to delay in diagnosis. Keratinocyte proliferation and vascular changes are the early features of EP in infants.[23]

Clinical Features

Erythroderma may arise from any type of psoriasis in children, but severe EP with joint and nail involvement is uncommon.The manifestations include erythema, desquamation, edema, fever, dehydration, malaise and malnutrition.[21]

Treatment

In severe and unstable cases: Cyclosporine or infliximab (due to their rapid action).

In milder cases: Methotrexate or acitretin.

Etanercept was the first biologic approved by the FDA (1999) for use in patients aged from 2 to 17 years with juvenile rheumatoid arthritis. Two patients with EP showed good response to etanercept.[22]

Prognosis

Erythroderma arising from any type of psoriasis in children is life-threatening leading to high morbidity and mortality. Correction of the hematologic, biochemical, and metabolic imbalance improves the final outcome.[21]

Future Perspectives[3]

Role of IL-23

IL-23 is an essential cytokine for differentiation of Th17 lymphocytes, which are implicated in the pathogenesis of psoriasis via production of pro-inflammatory cytokines such as IL-17A, IL-17F, and IL-22. IL-17A is considered a key 'driver' of proinflammatory cytokines in psoriasis pathogenesis since it can activate keratinocytes, causing hyper-proliferation and further production of antimicrobial peptides, cytokines, and chemokines, which, in turn, recruit and activate other immune cells, leading to amplification of psoriasis inflammation.

Evidence Supporting Role of IL-23

1. Mouse models of inflammation demonstrate that deficiency of IL-12 does not protect from the development of autoimmune diseases and these mice have a more severe clinical picture than their wild-type counterparts, hence it is possible to speculate a more important role for IL-23.

2. The messenger RNA (mRNA) levels of the subunit p19 (unique to IL-23) are elevated in psoriasis lesional skin compared with non-lesional skin, whereas the levels for p35 (a subunit distinct to IL-12) show no differences.

Clinical Implication of Role of IL-23

The newer/developmental anti-psoriatic biological agents targeting the IL-23/Th17 pathway might play a positive role in EP treatment.

These include:

- Tildrakizumab and guselkumab (targeting anti-IL-23 p19 antibodies)
- Secukinumab and ixekizumab (targeting anti-IL-17A antibodies)
- Brodalumab (an anti-IL-17-receptor antibody).

REFERENCES

1. Hawilo A, Zaraa I, Benmously R, Mebazaa A, El Euch D, Mokni M, Ben Osman A. Erythrodermic psoriasis: epidemiological clinical and therapeutic features about 60 cases. Tunis Med 2011;89(11):841–7.

2. Won-Ku Lee, Gun-Wook Kim, Hyun-Ho Cho, Won-Jeong Kim, Je-Ho Mun, Margaret Song, Hoon-Soo Kim, Hyun-Chang Ko, Moon-Bum Kim, 1,2 and Byung-Soo Kim. Erythrodermic Psoriasis Treated with Golimumab: A Case Report. Ann Dermatol 2015;27(4):446–9.

3. Giuseppe Stinco, Enzo Errichetti. Erythrodermic Psoriasis: Current and Future Role of Biologicals. BioDrugs 2015;29:91–101.

4. Rosita Saraceno,[a] Marina Talamonti,[a] Marco Galluzzo,[a] Andrea Chiricozzi,[a] Antonio Costanzo, and Sergio Chimentia. Ustekinumab

Treatment of Erythrodermic Psoriasis Occurring after Physical Stress: A Report of Two Cases. Case Rep Dermatol 2013;5(3):254–9.

5. Carlos G Teran, Carlos N Teran-Escalera, Carola Balderrama. A severe case of erythrodermic psoriasis associated with advanced nail and joint manifestations: a case report. J Med Case Reports 2010;4:179.

6. Wolfram Sterry, Chalid Assaf. Erythroderma, Dermatology, Jean L Bolognia, Joseph L Jorizzo, Ronald P Rapini (Eds). 2nd edn, vol 1, Mosby Elsevier, US. 2008;pp.149–58.

7. Chander Grover. Psoriasis. IADVL textbook of dermatology. Dr S Sacchidanand (Ed). 4th edn, Vol. 1, Bhalani publishing house, Mumbai, India. 2013, pp.1014–89.

8. Boyd AS, Menter A. Erythrodermic psoriasis. Precipitating factors, course, and prognosis in 50 patients. J Am Acad Dermatol 1989;21(5 Pt 1):985–91.

9. Wee JS, Natkunarajah J, Moosa Y, Marsden RA. Erythrodermic pustular psoriasis triggered by intravesical bacillus Calmette-Guérin immunotherapy. Clin Exp Dermatol 2012;37(4):455–7.

10. Cox NH, Gordon PM, Dodd H. Generalized pustular and erythrodermic psoriasis associated with bupropion treatment. Br J Dermatol 2002; 146(6):1061–3.

11. Evans AV, Parker JC, Russell-Jones R. Erythrodermic psoriasis precipitated by radiologic contrast media. J Am Acad Dermatol 2002; 46(6):960–1.

12. Pagliaro JA, Jones SK. Recurrent erythrodermic psoriasis in a thiuram-allergic patient due to contact with nurses' rubber gloves. Br J Dermatol 1999;140(3):567–8.

13. Zhang P, Chen HX, Duan YQ, Wang WZ, Zhang TZ, Li JW, Tu YT. Analysis of Th1/Th2 response pattern for erythrodermic psoriasis. J Huazhong Univ Sci Technolog Med Sci 2014;34(4):596–601.

14. Tomasini C, Aloi F, Solaroli C, Pippione M. Psoriatic erythroderma: a histopathologic study of forty-five patients. Dermatology 1997; 194(2):102–6.

15. Bruzzese V, Pepe J. Efficacy of cyclosporine in the treatment of a case of infliximab-induced erythrodermic psoriasis. Int J Immunopathol Pharmacol 2009;22(1):235–8.

16. Kokelj F, Plozzer C, Torsello P, Trevisan G. Efficacy of cyclosporine plus etretinate in the treatment of erythrodermic psoriasis (three case reports). J Eur Acad Dermatol Venereol 1998;11(2):177–9.

17. Geilen CC, Tebbe B, Garcia Bartels C, Krengel S, Orfanos CE. Successful treatment of erythrodermic psoriasis with mycophenolate mofetil. Br J Dermatol 1998;138(6):1101–2.

18. Arbiser JL, Grossman K, Kaye E, Arndt KA. Use of short-course class 1 topical glucocorticoid under occlusion for the rapid control of erythrodermic psoriasis. Arch Dermatol 1994;130(6):704–6.

19. Lekovixc B, Dostanic I, Konstantinovic K, Kneitner I. Treatment of pustulous and erythrodermic psoriasis with PUVA therapy and methotrexate. Hautarzt 1982;33(5):284–5.

20. Chiricozzi A, Saraceno R, Cannizzaro MV, Nisticò SP, Chimenti S, Giunta A. Complete resolution of erythrodermic psoriasis in an HIV and HCV patient unresponsive to antipsoriatic treatments after highly active antiretroviral therapy (Ritonavir, Atazanavir, Emtricitabine, Tenofovir). Dermatology 2012;225(4):333–7.

21. Jayashree Dinkar Patil, Shyam Sundar Chaudhary, Neha Rani, and Anup Kumar Mishra. Follicular psoriasis causing erythroderma in a child: A rare presentation Indian Dermatol Online J 2014;5(1):63–65.

22. Fraga NA, Paim Mde F, Follador I, Ramos AN, Rêgo VR. Refractory erythrodermic psoriasis in a child with an excellent outcome by using etanercept. An Bras Dermatol 2011;86(4 Suppl 1):S144–7.

23. Parimalam Kumar, Jayakar Thomas, Devaraj Dinesh Kumar. Histology of Psoriatic Erythroderma in Infants: Analytical Study of Eight Cases. Indian J Dermatol 2015;60(2):213.

5

Pediatric Psoriasis

Ragunatha S, Arun C Inamadar

Psoriasis is a chronic immune mediated papulosquamous disease predominantly occurring in adults. The recent epidemiological studies have shown that pediatric psoriasis is not uncommon. The diagnosis and management of pediatric psoriasis is challenging for various reasons. The clinical manifestations of psoriasis in children are atypical, leading to delay in identifying the disease by primary care physician. The current systemic therapy is not exact science as it is not evidence based. Hence, the children are repeatedly exposed to potential toxic drugs as they have to live with the disease longer than adults. In addition, the child is incapable of taking decision and depends on parents for everything, thus affecting quality of life of both child and parents. Hence, active participation of both treating physician and parents in understanding the nature of disease and various factors which determine course of the disease, and selection of appropriate management strategy is essential for desirable therapeutic outcome.

EPIDEMIOLOGY

The epidemiological data available on pediatric psoriasis is mainly derived from retrospective analysis of information. It is also hampered by the lack of clarity regarding case definition of psoriasis in children especially in infancy.[1] The upper limit of age set for pediatric group also differs among various studies.[1-5] The epidemiology varies among geographical areas because of difference in genetic susceptibility and predisposing factors. Hence, one has to be cautious before extrapolating the epidemiological data available in the literature.

Incidence and prevalence: The exact incidence of pediatric psoriasis is unknown. The annual incidence of pediatric psoriasis has increased from 29.6 cases per 100,000 in 1970 to 62.7 cases per 100,000 in 2000.[6] The worldwide prevalence ranges from 0.1 to 3%. In one third of adult patients with psoriasis, the onset of disease has been documented before the age of 16 years.[1,3] The pediatric psoriasis appears to be more common in clinical practice. They constitute 3.8 to 4.1% of all dermatoses seen in children below 16 years in Turkey[3] and Europe and North America[7] respectively. Whereas in North India, psoriasis constituted 0.3%[5] and in South India 1.4%[4] of all pediatric dermatoses. In North India, the point prevalence of psoriasis in the age group of 6–14 years was found to be 0.02%.[8] Psoriatic arthritis (PsA) is very rare in children and constitutes 0[1,3] to 4%[2] of pediatric psoriasis cases.

Age distribution: The prevalence of the disease in children increases linearly from 0.09% at one year to 0.82% at 18 years.[9] The peak age of onset of psoriasis is varied in different studies owing to varied clinical case definition of psoriasis and omission of certain types like diaper rash or scalp-only involvement from some of the studies. Based on age of onset, pediatric psoriasis can be categorized arbitrarily as congenital below 2 years, 2–9 years (pre-pubertal) and >10 years (pubertal). In congenital psoriasis, the lesions appear at birth or within a few days. It is very rare. The proportion of children with psoriasis below one year and two years of age has been reported to be 6.25[10] to 16%[1] and 6[11] to 27%[1] respectively. In 56% of children, the disease manifests during pre-pubertal age.[2] A bimodal age of onset of PsA has been described. Early onset form peaks during the first few years and adolescenct form peaks during early adolescence.[12]

Gender distribution: The pediatric psoriasis seems to be slightly common in girls, though studies from India[10] and Australia[1] have showed equal gender distribution. Regarding age of patients or age of onset of disease there has been no significant difference between the genders.[3] However, certain clinical types of psoriasis demonstrate male or female preponderance. Scalp-only psoriasis[1] and early onset PsA are more common in girls and genital involvement[2] and adolescent onset PsA[13] in pre-pubertal boys.

Predisposing factors: Generally, unlike adults, children are at increased risk of trauma and recurrent infections. Hence, upper respiratory tract infections (URTI), positive throat culture, stress and psychiatric morbidity are common predisposing factors recognized in 14.8%, 21.3%, 54% and 9.8% of patients with pediatric psoriasis respectively. Though URTI is the well-known predisposing factor for guttate psoriasis, a positive throat culture, stress and psychiatric morbidities are commonly associated with pustular psoriasis when compared to other clinical types.[3] The analysis of environmental risk factors has demonstrated possible role of high body mass index (BMI), exposure to smoking at home and stressful life events in the development of pediatric psoriasis.[14]

Family history: The positive family history ranges from 4.5% to 91%. In majority of cases, the first-degree relatives were affected. The frequency of family history of psoriasis is related to age of onset of disease; with increase in age at onset of psoriasis the detection of family history of disease increases.[3] In India, the relatively low frequency of family history (4.5 to 9.8%) can be attributed to ignorance about the disease, non-disclosure due to social reasons or actual absence at the time of enquiry.[15]

Ethnic variation: The ethnic differences in epidemiology of pediatric psoriasis in European (Dutch) and Asian (Singapore) children has revealed significantly higher positive family history, symptoms (itching) and predisposing factors in Dutch children. The gender distribution, age of onset, site of involvement and type of psoriasis were similar in both ethnic groups.[16]

Genetic susceptibility: The early onset psoriasis (<40 years) is associated with HLA Cw6 allele. It is associated with pubertal age of onset, guttate psoriasis and facial involvement.[2]

Quality of life: Pediatric psoriasis negatively affects the physical, emotional and social functioning of children irrespective of severity of the disease. It is worse than children with diabetes and epilepsy. Even in mild psoriasis, the stigmatization reported in 65%, itching in 71% and fatigue in 43% of children. Quality of life issue is important because of lack of coping mechanisms in younger children.[17]

ETIOPATHOGENESIS

Psoriasis is characterized by T cell mediated autoimmune response against self-antigen. The increased rate of positive family history and infections in pediatric psoriasis indicate role of genetic susceptibility and environmental factors in the development of disease. Hence, psoriasis appears to be a result of autoimmune response against unknown self-antigen triggered by an environmental factor in a genetically susceptible individual. The pathogenic process involving various immune cells, cytokines and growth factors is similar to that of adults and detailed description of complex interplay between host immune response and environmental factors is out of scope of this chapter.[18]

Clinical Features

In general, the psoriatic lesions are thinner, less scaly and more pruritic in children posing diagnostic dilemma especially in children < two years of age (Figs 5.1 and 5.2). In dark-skinned children, the scales are so subtle that the lesions present as hypopigmented patches showing scales only on scratching.[1] Plaque psoriasis remains the commonest clinical variant irrespective of age of children. However, involvement of diaper area, flexures, face and anogenital area is unique and can be sole manifestations in children.[1–3] Pityriasis amiantacea characterized by asbestos like scales encircling tuft of hairs on scalp is particularly observed in children (Fig. 5.3). Majority of these cases show staphylococcal overgrowth which may act as triggering factor in causation of disease.[19] The characteristic physical findings of psoriasis like Auspitz sign, Koebner phenomenon and postinflammatory pigmentary changes are also seen in pediatric psoriasis.[18] The morphology of the lesions, site of involvement, severity of the disease and course and prognosis are varied in different pediatric age groups.

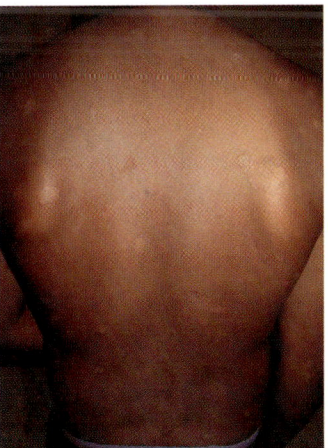 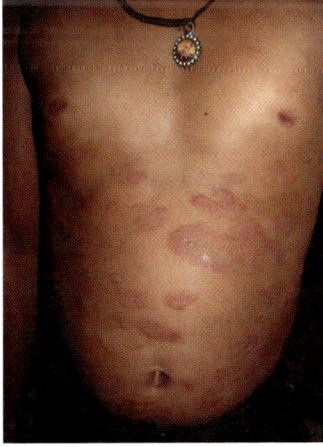

Figs 5.1 and 5.2 Thinner and less scaly psoriatic lesions in children

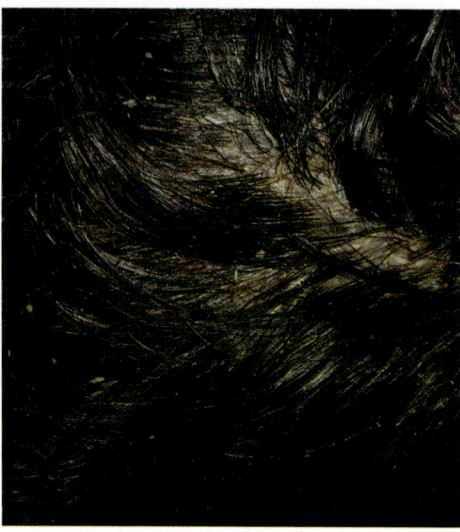

Fig. 5.3 Asbestos like scales on the scalp in pityriasis amiantacea

Congenital psoriasis: The commonest clinical variants of congenital psoriasis are plaque, erythrodermic and pustular psoriasis. Linear psoriasis along the Blashko's line has been reported. The lesions usually involve scalp, extremities, trunk and face. The diaper area is spared due to absence of irritation and occlusion in diaper-naïve newborns. The clinical variants of congenital psoriasis tend to be more severe with poor prognosis compared to infantile and childhood psoriasis. This observation is associated with publication bias, as mild cases are either underreported or misdiagnosed.[20]

Below 2 years: The involvement of diaper area is unique in children below 2 years. The disease is either localized to diaper area or associated with dissemination. After exclusion of diaper rash psoriasis, plaque, acropustulosis and guttate type are the commonest variants in this age group. The diaper rash in psoriasis is bright red, well demarcated and shinier than seborrheic dermatitis. In majority of patients, the course of the disease is mild.[1]

Between 2 and 9 years: Flexural (inverse), anogenital and facial involvement is characteristic in this age group. Groin, axillae and retroauricular area are involved in inverse psoriasis (Figs 5.4 to 5.6). The presence of lesions on genitalia (Fig. 5.7) and around the eye is distinguishing feature that helps in the differential diagnosis of atypical cases.[2]

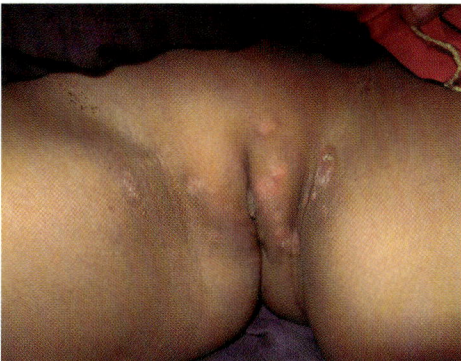

Fig. 5.4 Erythematous scaly plaque involving groin in inverse psoriasis

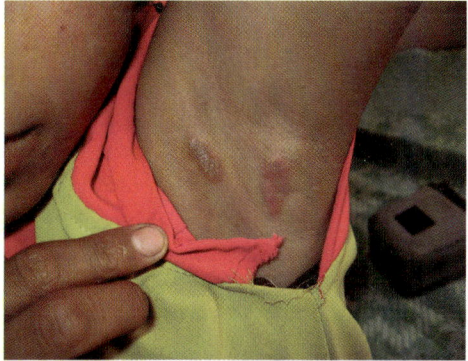

Fig. 5.5 Erythematous scaly plaque involving axilla in inverse psoriasis

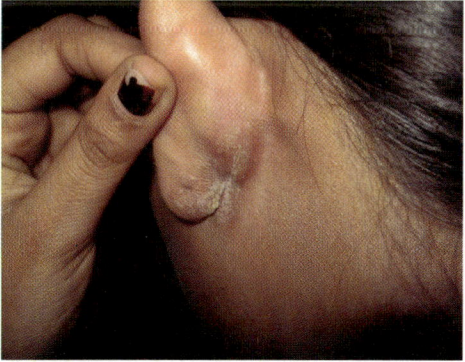

Fig. 5.6 Erythematous scaly plaque involving retroauricular area in inverse psoriasis

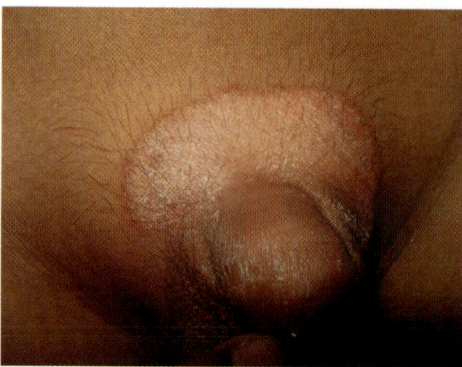

Fig. 5.7 Erythematous scaly plaque involving genitalia

>10 years: The occurrence of guttate psoriasis is common though other clinical variants occur with less frequency when compared to other age groups. Guttate psoriasis is characterized by sudden eruption of erythematous plaques measuring 0.5 to 1 cm with scales distributed over trunk, face and extremities (Fig. 5.8).[21] Usually, the guttate psoriasis resolves completely without recurrences, but in some cases may progress to chronic plaque psoriasis.[22]

Nail involvement: Nail pitting can be the first sign of disease in 2% of pediatric psoriasis.[23] Nail changes occur in almost one-third of patients. These include pitting, subungual hyperkeratosis, longitudinal striae, discoloration and onycholysis.[2]

Mucosal involvement: Erythematous patches on oral or genital mucosa, oral erosions and geographic tongue has been reported in 5.6% of children with psoriasis.[23] Geographic tongue can occur in 3.3% of cases.[2]

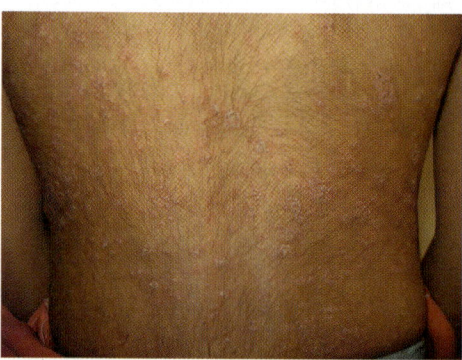

Fig. 5.8 Erythematous plaques measuring 0.5 to 1 cm with scales distributed over trunk in guttate psoriasis

Rare variants: Erythrodermic, pustular, linear, palmoplantar and follicular variants are rare in children.[1] Pustular psoriasis can be generalized or localized, the latter being extremely rare in children.[3] Generalized pustular psoriasis is slightly common in boys. It is generally associated with malaise, fever and anorexia, but runs a benign course in children compared to adults. In infants, von Zumbusch type is more common and pustular psoriasis occurs *de novo*. However, in 30% of cases history of seborrheic dermatitis or napkin dermatitis can be elicited.[21] Later in childhood, annular pattern and mixed pattern appear.[24]

PsA is inflammatory seronegative arthritis which may precede, coincide or follow skin lesions.[21] It is preceded by skin lesions in 80% of patients. In early stage, oligoarthritis is commonly seen involving distal and proximal interphalangeal (IP) joints of feet, IP joints of hand, knees and ankles. In later stages, wrist, elbow, metacarpophalangeal and metatarsophalangeal joints are affected. Bluish discoloration over affected joints when present is a distinguishing feature of PsA.[25]

Comorbidity: Association of psoriasis with metabolic syndrome and cardiovascular diseases in adults is well known. Some studies demonstrated increased rate of hypertension, hyperlipidemia, diabetes mellitus and obesity in children with psoriasis compared to healthy controls.[26] However, the onset of psoriasis in childhood is not associated with increased risk of cardiovascular disease and metabolic syndrome in adulthood. Severity of disease is associated with obesity and increased risk of smoking.[27]

Clinical course: Pediatric psoriasis usually runs a benign course though there is no consensus whether early onset of disease predicts milder or more severe form of psoriasis. Generally, the severity of disease diminishes but the clinical type remains the same with advancing age. However, pediatric psoriasis is associated with increased frequency of guttate and erythrodermic psoriasis in adulthood.[28]

Differential Diagnosis

Atypical nature of clinical manifestations and distinctive site of predilection makes pediatric psoriasis a diagnostic challenge. Various papulosquamous, infectious, allergic and immunological diseases need to be considered in the differential diagnosis depending on clinical type of psoriasis (Table 5.1).[18]

Table 5.1: Differential diagnosis of common clinical variants of pediatric psoriasis[18]

Clinical type	Differential diagnosis	Diagnostic features	Investigations
Inverse psoriasis	Seborrheic dermatitis	Yellow greasy scales, less demarcated and less shinier than psoriasis	Skin biopsy
	Candidiasis	Macerated erythematous plaques with satellite pustules	KOH preparation
	Contact dermatitis	Sparing of inguinal folds	Skin biopsy
	Dermatophytoses	Annular papules with peripheral scaling and central clearing	KOH preparation
	Erythrasma	Uniformly pigmented, well-demarcated brown patch	Coral red fluorescence on Wood's lamp
	Langerhans' cell histiocytosis	Crusting and scaling with hemorrhagic papules with lymphadenopathy	Skin biopsy and immunohistochemistry
Guttate psoriasis	Pityriasis rosea	Herald patch, knee-elbow distribution and christmas tree pattern	Skin biopsy
	Pityriasis lichenoideschronica	Reddish-brown papules with micaceous small scales, recurrent crops	Skin biopsy
	Secondary syphilis	Involvement of palms and soles, Ollendorff sign	VDRL, TPHA

Contd...

Table 5.1: Differential diagnosis of common clinical variants of pediatric psoriasis[18] (Contd...)

Clinical type	Differential diagnosis	Diagnostic features	Investigations
Generalized plaque psoriasis	Pityriasis rosea	Herald patch, collarette scales and christmas tree pattern	Skin biopsy
	Small plaque parapsoriasis	Thin less erythematous or hypopigmented plaques with fine scaling	Skin biopsy
	Lichen planus	Pruritic, flat topped, polygonal, violaceous papules on flexor aspect of extremities	Skin biopsy
	Subacute cutaneous lupus erythematosus	Annular lesions with photosensitivity	Skin biopsy
	Extensive dermatophytoses	Annular papules with peripheral scaling and central clearing	KOH preparation
	Type 1 lepra reaction	Preexisting hypopigmented patches, tenderness of lesions, enlarged peripheral nerves	Skin biopsy, slit skin smear
	Secondary syphilis	Involvement of palms and soles	VDRL, TPHA
	Pityriasis rubra pilaris	Follicular papules with interfollicular erythema and bran like scales involving	Skin biopsy

Contd...

Table 5.1: Differential diagnosis of common clinical variants of pediatric psoriasis[18] (Contd...)

Clinical type	Differential diagnosis	Diagnostic features	Investigations
		scalp. Involvement of proximal phalynx, island of normal skin, and kerato-dermic sandal like palms and soles are characteristic	
Scalp psoriasis	Tinea capitis	Broken and easily pluckable hairs with occipital lymphadenopathy	Wood's lamp, KOH preparation
	Seborrheic dermatitis	Diffuse involvement with yellow greasy scales	Skin biopsy
	Discoid lupus erythematoses	Scarring alopecia with depigmentation	Skin biopsy
Psoriatic arthritis	Juvenile rheumatoid arthritis	Bluish discoloration of joints, nail changes and predominant involvement of wrist and small joints of hands and feet favor diagnosis of psoriatic arthritis	RA factor, antinuclear antibodies, radiography

Note: KOH, Potassium hydroxide; TPHA, Treponema pallidum hemagglutination test; VDRL, Veneral Disease Research Laboratory

Diagnosis and Laboratory Evaluation

In atypical cases skin biopsy and relevant investigations (*see* Table 5.1) help in differential diagnosis. The histopathology shows diagnostic epidermal and dermal changes similar to adult psoriasis. Continuous laboratory evaluation at regular interval is important to identify predisposing factors, comorbid conditions and adverse effects of drugs.[18]

Management

In general, the management of pediatric psoriasis is conservative because of less severe and milder course of the disease. The long term safety data on drugs and evidence based therapy in pediatric psoriasis is limited. Hence, the dermatologists need to depend on experience and extrapolation of results from treatment of psoriasis in adults. As the child requires long-term therapy, an individually tailored management strategy should be evolved by involving children and parents in decision making.[29]

For optimal therapeutic outcome, evaluation of factors which determine choice of therapy (Table 5.2) and strategic use of topical and systemic drugs to maximize the benefits and minimize cumulative toxicities of drugs (Table 5.3) is essential.[29]

Specific Drug Therapy for Psoriasis

Majority of drugs either topical or systemic that are tried and tested in adult psoriasis are used in the treatment of pediatric psoriasis. The pattern of prescription by dermatologists for pediatric psoriasis showed predominant use of topical corticosteroids (91.2%)

Table 5.2: Determinants of choice of therapy

- Age of the patient
- Primary morphology (pustular/guttate/erythroderma/plaque)
- Progression of disease (rapidly evolving/chronic)
- Severity of disease
- Concern about specific symptom of disease
- Comorbidity and triggers
- Impact on quality of life
- Family history of psoriasis
- Involvement of joints
- Experience of dermatologist in particular therapy/drug
- Cost-effectiveness

Table 5.3: Strategic use of drugs in pediatric psoriasis

Combination therapy: A lower dosage of each agents is used. After the clearance of psoriasis usually one agent is discontinued and the safer of the two is used as maintenance therapy. Indications of combination therapy include failure of monotherapy, emergence of toxicity to single agent, when potentially toxic drugs are to be used, and tapering the patient from an individual drug.

Rotational therapy: Different treatment regimens are rotated before significant toxicity to individual drug develops. The therapeutic agent is used for specified period (usually 1–2 years) after which alternative drug is started. It allows long-term treatment and minimum chronic toxicity.

Sequential therapy:
- *Clearing phase*: Initially, a rapidly acting but potentially more toxic agent is used at a maximum dose to clear the psoriasis.
- *Transition phase*: A weaker less toxic agent is introduced while gradually tapering the initial drug to maintain the clearance.
- *Maintenance phase*: Only maintenance drug is continued as long as required with or without UVB or PUVA.

followed by vitamin D analogues (73.5%), phototherapy (64.7%), systemic drugs (20.6%), dithranol (20.6%) and coal tar (11.8%).[30]

Topical preparations: In mild to moderate psoriasis, topical therapy either alone or in combination with other topical and systemic drugs is mainstay of treatment. Moisturizers and keratolytics are considered as basic therapy in psoriasis. The former decreases scaling, limits painful fissuring and is anti-pruritic. Topical keratolytics like salicylic acid are used in case of thick scales and palmoplantar lesions. Salicylic acid should not be applied if body surface area involved in >20%.[31] Among all intended to treat topical drugs, corticosteroids and calcipotriol are evaluated for safety and efficacy. The choice of topical agent depends on site of involvement, morphology of lesions, irritant potential, long-term side effects and cosmetic acceptability (Table 5.4).[21,25,31]

Systemic therapy: During the course of disease the child may experience severe and debilitating episodes. The presence of pustular lesions, erythroderma, rapidly evolving disease, low quality of life, positive family history and involvement of joints indicate severe and chronic course requiring systemic drugs (Table 5.5). In children, it is mainly empirical because none of the agents are approved for use below 18 years owing to limited

Table 5.4: Topical therapy in pediatric psoriasis[18,21,25,31]

Topical preparation	Mode of action	Usage	Limitations and concerns	Role in treatment strategy
Topical corticosteroids	Antiproliferative, anti-inflammatory	Treatment of choice for flexural disease and recommended for face and scalp lesions. Preferred in itching lesions	Tachyphylaxis and cutaneous side effects like striae and telengectasia. Use least potent agent for shortest possible time	Monotherapy or combination therapy with calcipotriol, salicylic acid, PUVA and systemic agents
Vitamin D analogues	Antiproliferative, promotion of epidermal differentiation, anti-inflammatory	Effective and well tolerated in the treatment of pediatric psoriasis. Maximum dose up to 50 mg/week for children >6 years and 75 mg/week for children >12 years	Effect on calcium metabolism. Monitoring of serum calcium in case of long-term use. Report of facial irritation in a few patients. Should be applied after phototherapy	Monotherapy or combination therapy with topical corticosteroids PUVA and systemic agents
Coal tar	Antiproliferative and antipruritic	Suitable for use on face and genitals as it is less irritant. Used in plaque and guttate psoriasis	Unpleasant smell and tendency to stain. Concerns about carcinogenicity of coal tar	Combination therapy with UVB in Goekerman regimen

Contd...

Table 5.4: Topical therapy in pediatric psoriasis[18,21,25,31] (Contd...)

Topical preparation	Mode of action	Usage	Limitations and concerns	Role in treatment strategy
Dithranol	Antiproliferative	Useful on thick plaques with a large surface area.	Irritation and staining of healthy skin. Not suitable for face, genitalia and flexures. Should be avoided in pustular and erythrodermic psoriasis	Short contact for 30 to 40 min at low concentration (0.1 to 0.25%) and slowly increase to 2 to 3% as tolerance develops
Calcineurin inhibitors	Immunosuppressants	Effective on face, flexures and genital lesions. Tacrolimus (0.03% in children 2–15 years and 0.1% in children >16 years) and pimecrolimus 1% are off-label indications in psoriasis	Burning at the site of application.	Used as monotherapy
Tazarotene 0.1%	Normalizes abnormal proliferation and differentiation	Effective in nail and palmoplantar psoriasis.	Perilesional skin irritation In sensitive skin use 0.05% cream, alternate day treatment and short contact for 5 minutes	Combination with topical corticosteroids gives superior result

Note: PUVA, Psoralen Ultraviolet A therapy; UVB, Ultraviolet B

Table 5.5: Systemic therapy in pediatric psoriasis[21,25,31]

Drugs	Dosage and indications	Strategic usage	Caution
Methotrexate	Dosage: 0.2–0.7mg/kg per week Indications: Moderate to severe psoriasis, palmoplantar psoriasis, recalcitrant psoriasis, erythroderma, pustular psoriasis and psoriatic arthritis	Ideal for clearing (rescue) phase of sequential therapy. Also used as monotherapy and with other agents in combination or rotation therapy.	Avoid concomitant use of sulphonamides and NSAIDs due to risk of life threatening bone marrow toxicity during first 4–6 wks. Pulmonary and hepatic toxicity is rare in children.
Phototherapy	Indications: Guttate psoriasis (responds best), extensive body surface area involvement, refractory psoriasis to topical combination therapy, contraindications to systemic agents, debilitating palmoplantar psoriasis	Combination of NBUVB with coal tar in Goekerman regimen. Combination of NBUVB with topicals like calcipotriene, tazarotene and anthralin.	Avoid psoralens in children below 12 years due to risk of cutaneous carcinogenesis
Acitretin	Dosage: 0.5 to 1 mg/kg per day Indications: Pustular, guttate, erythrodermic and palmoplantar psoriasis	Clearing phase of sequential therapy for generalized pustular psoriasis. Alone or in combination with NBUVB during maintenance phase for pustular, erythrodermic, severe guttate, severe plaque psoriasis. Rotation therapy as cyclic short term use for 6 to 12 months	Avoid supplements containing >5000 IU of vitamin A, long-term (>1 year) uninterrupted use in pre-pubertal children and pregnancy during and for 3 years after stopping acitretin. Mucocutaneous side effects are common at doses near 1 mg/kg/day

Contd...

Table 5.5: Systemic therapy in pediatric psoriasis[21,25,31] *(Contd...)*

Drugs	Dosage and indications	Strategic usage	Caution
Cyclosporine	Dosage: 1.5–5 mg/kg per day. Indications: Rapidly evolving or recalcitrant plaque psoriasis, pustular psoriasis. Starting dose is 5 mg/kg/day in severe and debilitating psoriasis followed by slow tapering	Clearing phase of sequential therapy for severe, rapidly evolving and debilitating disease. Combination with acitretin or topical agents	Combination with NBUVB not preferred due to risk of squamous cell carcinoma though it is minimal at doses <5 mg/kg/day. Avoid live attenuated vaccines. Vaccination may be less effective. Avoid continuous use for >1 to 2 yrs.
Biologicals	Dosage: Etanercept: 0.8 mg/kg weekly subcutaneously Infliximab: 3.3–5 mg/kg intravenously at week 0, 2, 6 and then then every 7–8 weeks Adalimumab: 24 mg/m² subcutaneously (maximum 40 mg) every 2 wks Ustekinumab: Not specified, has been used at a dose of 45 mg subcutaneous at 0 and 4 weeks and then every 12 wks Indications: Second or third line therapy for recalcitrant plaque, erythrodermic, pustular or palmoplantar psoriasis, and psoriatic arthritis	Clearing phase of sequential therapy	Black box warning for risk of lymphoma and other cancers in children taking TNF-α inhibitors. Avoid live and live attenuated vaccines.

Note: NBUVB, Narrow Band Ultraviolet B therapy; NSAIDs, Non-steroidal Anti-inflammatory Drugs

evidences on efficacy and long-term safety data. The children usually tolerate systemic drugs like acitretin and cyclosporine better than adults. Safety and efficacy of these drugs has been established in children treated for disorders of keratinization and atopic dermatitis respectively. In pediatric psoriasis, acitretin and cyclosporine have been used successfully in children as young as 6 months and 11 months respectively. Similarly, methotrexate has been used safely in children between 2 and 16 years with psoriasis. However, careful monitoring of adverse effects and laboratory parameters as in adults is recommended when these drugs are intended to use for longer period of time.[29]

In majority of patients with recalcitrant pediatric psoriasis the order of switch from previously failed therapy to next therapy has been topicals to methotrexate or phototherapy, phototherapy to methotrexate or etanercept, methotrexate to etanercept or cyclosporine, cyclosporine to etanercept, etanercept to adalimumab, and finally adalimumab to ustekinumab.[32] Etanercept is the only biological therapy with established safety and efficacy through randomized controlled study. It is the preferred second line of therapy in recalcitrant pediatric psoriasis. Biologicals have a potential of ideal first line treatment option for pediatric psoriasis because of less frequent dosing and laboratory monitoring and absence of serious end-organ toxicities in comparison to conventional systemic agents.[29]

Adjuvant Therapy

Adjuvant therapy like maintenance of barrier function, treatment of predisposing factors and comorbidity, symptomatic treatment, nutritional supplementation and parental counselling is essential to maximize the effectiveness of specific treatment of psoriasis.

Antistreptococcal antibiotic and tonsillectomy: Streptococcal infection is a well-known predisposing factor. Several studies have implicated subclinical or recurrent streptococcal infection as trigger or maintenance factor in the pathogenesis of psoriasis. Treatment with antistreptococcal antibiotics and tonsillectomy appears to be an effective adjuvant therapy. However, such therapy remains controversial. Randomized controlled trials have failed to show their efficacy in the treatment of psoriasis.[33]

Parental counselling: The successful implementation of management strategy depends on attitude of parents as their involvement and cooperation is must for compliance. Parental motivation is very important because taking care of child with psoriasis also affects their quality of life. Hence, the treatment should be simple and practical without interfering with routine activities of child and/or parents.[21,25]

Symptomatic treatment: The symptom of disease which causes most distress needs to be addressed immediately with appropriate intervention. Some children are concerned only about scaling, whereas others worry about itching and older children and adolescents are anxious about cosmetic aspects.[21]

Nutritional supplementation: In severe and erythrodermic forms of psoriasis, significant amount of fluid and nutrition is lost. Transepidermal water loss occurs through damaged skin barrier and protein and iron is lost through exfoliated skin. Hence, supplementation of fluid and nutrition is very important to maintain normal hemodynamic state and metabolic functions of the body.[34]

Laser therapy: Excimer laser (308 nm) has been used successfully in the treatment of localized psoriasis affecting palms, soles, scalp, face and other parts of body. It is generally well tolerated by children.[18]

REFERENCES

1. Morris A, Rogers M, Fisher G, Williams K. Childhood psoriasis: A clinical review of 1262 cases. Pediatr Dermatol 2008;18:188–98.
2. Lysell J, Tessma M, Nikamo P, Wahlgren C, Stahle M. Clinical characterization at the onset of childhood psoriasis: A cross-sectional study in Sweden. ActaDermVenereol 2015;95:457–61.
3. Seyhan M, Coskun BK, Saglam H, Ozcan H, Karincaoglu Y. Psoriasis in childhood and adolescence: Evaluation of demographic and clinical features. Pediatrics International 2006;48:525–30.
4. Karthikeyan K, Thappa DM, Jeevankumar B. Pattern of pediatric dermatoses in a referral center in South India. Indian Pediatr 2004; 41: 373–7.
5. Kumar B, Jain R, Sandhu K, Kumar B. Epidemiology of childhood psoriasis: A study of 419 patients from northern India. Int J Dermatol 2004;43:654–8.
6. Tollefson MM, Crowson CS, McEvoy MT, Maradit Kremers H. Incidence of psoriasis in children: A population-based study. J Am Acad Dermatol 2010;62:979–87.

7. Marcoux D, de Prost Y. Pediatric psoriasis revisited. J Cutan Med Surg 2002;6:22–8.

8. Dogra S, Kumar B. Epidemiology of skin diseases in school children: A study from Northern India. PediatrDermatol 2003;20:470–3.

9. Matusiewicz D, Koerber A, Schadendorf D, Wasem J, Neumann A. Childhood Psoriasis—An Analysis of German Health Insurance Data. 2014;31:18–13.

10. Nanda A, Kaur S, Kaur I, Kumar B. Childhood psoriasis: An epidemiological survey of 112 patients. Pediatr Dermatol 1990;7:19–21.

11. Nyfors A, Lemholt K. Psoriasis in children: a short review of 245 cases. Br J Dermatol 1975;92:437–42.

12. Stoll ML, Nigrovic PA. Subpopulations within juvenile psoriatic arthritis: a review of literature. Clin Dev Immunol 2006;13:377–80.

13. Stoll ML, Punaro M. Psoriatic juvenile idiopathic arthritis: a tale of two subgroups. Curr Opin Rheumatol 2011;23:437–43.

14. Ozden MG, Tekin NS, Gurer MA, Akdemir D, Dogramaci C, Utas S, et al. Environmental risk factors in pediatric psoriasis: A multicentre case-control study. Pediatric Dermatology 2011;28:306–12.

15. Dogra S, Kaur I. Childhood psoriasis. Indian J Dermatol Venereol Leprol 2010;76:357–65.

16. Chiam LYT, de Jager MEA, Giam YC, de Jong EMGJ, van de Kerkhof PCM, Seyger MMB. Juvenile psoriasis in European and Asian children: similarities and differences. Br J Dermatol 2011;164:1101–03.

17. deJager MEA, de Jong EMGJ, Evers AWM, van de Kerkhof PCM, Seyger MMB. Burden of childhood psoriasis. Pediatr Dermatol 2011; 28:736–7.

18. Pepper AN, Pothiawala S, Silverberg NB. Pediatric psoriasis. In: Weinberg JM, Lebwohl M, (Eds). Advances in psoriasis London: Springer 2014, p 253–76.

19. Abdel-Hamid AI, Agha SA, Moustafa YM, El-Labban AM. Pityriasis amiantacia: a clinical and etiological study of 85 patients. Int J dermatol 2003;42:260–4.

20. Lehman JS, Rahil AK. Congenital psoriasis: case report and literature review. PediatrDermatol 2008;25:232–8.

21. Leman J, Burden D. Psoriasis in children. A guide to its diagnosis and management. Paediatr Drugs 2001;3:673–80.

22. Martin BA, Chalmers RJG, Telfer NR, et al. How great is the risk of further psoriasis following a single episode of acute guttate psoriasis? Arch Dermatol 1996;132:717–8.

23. Nanda A, Al-Fouzan AS, El-Kashlan M, Al-Sweih N, Al-Muzairai I. Salient features and HLA markers of childhood psoriasis in Kuwait. Clin. Exp. Dermatol 2000;25:147–51.

24. Burden AD. Management of psoriasis in childhood. Clin Exp Dermatol 199;24:341–5.

25. Lewkowicz D, Gottleib AB. Pediatric psoriasis and psoriatic arthritis. Dermatologic Therapy 2004;17:364–75.

26. Augustin M, Glaeske G, Radtke MA, et al. Epidemiology and comorbidity of psoriasis in children. Br J Dermatol 2010;162:633–6.

27. Mahe E, Maccari F, Beauchet A, Lahfa M, Barthelemy H, Reguiai Z, et al. Childhood-onset psoriasis: Association with future cardiovascular and metabolic comorbidities. Br J Dermatol 2013;169:889–95.

28. deJager MEA, de Jong EMGJ, Meeuwis KAP, van de Kerkhof PCM, Seyger MMB. No evidence found that childhood onset of psoriasis influences disease severity, future body mass index or type of treatments used. J Euro Acad Dermatol Venereol 2010;24:1333–9.

29. Marqueling AL, Cordoro KM. Systemic treatments for severe pediatric psoriasis. A practical approach. Dermatol Clin 2013;31:267–88.

30. deJager MEA, van de Kerkhof PCM, de Jong EMGJ, Seyger MMB. Epidemiology and prescribed treatments in childhood psoriasis: A survey among medical professionals. J Dermatol Treat 2009;20:254–8.

31. Guenther LC. Topical Therapy II: Retinoids, immunomodulators, and others. In: Weinberg JM, Lebwohl M, (Eds). Advances in psoriasis. London: Springer 2014, p.73–89.

32. Garber C, Creighton-Smith M, Sorensen EP, Dumont N, Gottleib AB. Systemic treatment of recalcitrant pediatric psoriasis: A case series and literature review. J Drug Dermatol 2015;14:881–7.

33. Wilson JK, Al-Suwaidan SN, Krowchuk D, Feldman SR. Treatment of psoriasis in childhood: Is there a role for antibiotic therapy and tonsillectomy? Pediatr Dermatol 2003;20:11–5.

34. Ragunatha S, Inamadar AC. Neonatal dermatological emergencies. Indian J Dermatol Venereol Leprol 2010;76:328–40.

6

Psoriasis in Pregnancy

Parag Chaudhari

INTRODUCTION

The prevalence of psoriasis ranges from 0.1 to 3% as reported from various studies. It is not infrequent to encounter psoriasis in pregnancy. Various forms of clinical presentations of the disease are seen in pregnancy. Effect on fetus may occur due to psoriasis or medications used for treatment. It is important for physician to be aware of the drugs that can be used as well as those which are contraindicated during pregnancy or lactation.

The effect of pregnancy on psoriasis is variable. Pregnancy may influence the severity of psoriasis. In fact, psoriasis often improves during pregnancy. The alterations in immunity from Th1 to Th2 dominance due to hormonal changes in pregnancy leads to the improvement in psoriasis.[1] These females subsequently develop a "post-partum flare" of their psoriasis. Interleukin-10 (IL-10) levels are raised in pregnancy.[2] It has anti-inflammatory and immune suppressive effect which may be responsible for improvement in psoriasis.

On the other hand, some females may experience exacerbation of psoriasis. This exacerbation usually recurs in subsequent pregnancies.

Pregnancy can act as precipitating factor for development of erythrodermic or pustular psoriasis. Pregnancy may act as a triggering factor for the articular disease and psoriatic arthritis can occur in post-partum period.[3]

Placental vasculopathy in mothers suffering from psoriasis can cause intrauterine growth retardation and low birth weight.[4, 5] Also, psoriasis is associated with high rates of comorbidities, such as diabetes mellitus, cardiovascular diseases, obesity and metabolic syndrome that may also lead to complications during pregnancy and increase the risk of malformations. It should also be kept in mind that fetus may be affected by medications that are used for psoriasis.

Impetigo herpetiformis:[6] It is characteristic form of pustular psoriasis seen in pregnancy. It commonly occurs in third trimester. It can be associated with hypocalcemia and hypoparathyroidism. Erythematous plaques appear initially in flexures. The pustules appear at periphery of plaques. Centrifugal spread occurs to involve entire body relatively sparing face, hands and feet. It is accompanied by fever, dehydration and tachycardia. The condition tends to improve postpartum. There is risk of recurrence with even higher severity in subsequent pregnancies. The differential diagnosis include erythema multiforme, dermatitis herpeteformis and subconeal pustular dermatosis. The treatment of choice is systemic corticosteroids with daily 30–60 mg of prednisone in tapering doses. Cyclosporin may be used in refractory cases. Correction of hypocalcemia is required along with fluids and electrolytes management.

MANAGEMENT OF PSORIASIS IN PREGNANCY

Topical treatment is the first-line treatment of psoriasis in pregnant and lactating women. Emollients should be added to low to medium potency corticosteroids due to lack of adverse effects. Percutaneous absorption of corticosteroids depends on dose, excipient, treatment surface and application site, treatment duration, use of occlusive dressings and frequency of applications. It is useful to advise the patient not to apply excessive amounts over large areas, or on those under occlusion, to avoid excessive absorption and possible risk of low birth weight.[3,7]

Phototherapy with broadband (290–320 nm) ultraviolet B (UVB) and narrowband UVB (311–312 nm) appear to be safe during pregnancy. It was not associated with increased risk of fetal abnormalities or prematurity though data is limited. It is preferred for treatment for extensive disease.

PUVA therapy constitutes use of psoralens with ultraviolet light. It is not recommended due to mutagenicity although some consider topical PUVA safe.

Tacrolimus has been used to treat psoriasis on face as well as intertriginous areas. There are no adequate studies on the use of topical tacrolimus during pregnancy. The advantages are lack of skin atrophy and it is absorbed percutaneously to lesser extent compared to steroids.

Treatment with topical salicylic acid is controversial. No studies have been published on the use of topical salicylic acid in pregnant women.

Other agents like anthralin, coal tar, calcipotriol vitamin D_3 analogue are used topically in psoriasis. However, these are generally not preferred due to lack of proven safety and limited data is available.

Tazarotene is not used in pregnancy due to risk of teratogenicity—fetal death and malformations found in animal studies.

Systemic corticosteroids are not routinely used in the treatment of psoriasis. Although their use is associated with rapid clearing of lesions, exacerbation occurs after stopping. They are indicated in erythroderma unresponsive to other therapies and fulminant generalized pustular psoriasis when other drugs are ineffective or contraindicated.

The use of cyclosporine showed no increased risk to the fetus and may be an option in psoriasis. It can be considered in extensive disease not responding to topical therapy and UVB phototherapy. The disadvantages are adverse effects like hypertension and nephrotoxicity which can complicate pregnancy.

Methotrexate can cause growth retardation, spontaneous miscarriage, cleft palate and other skeletal abnormalities. Hence it is absolutely contraindiacted in pregnancy.[8]

Acetretin and systemic retinoid can cause cardiac, craniofacial and central nervous system malformations and thus are contraindicated during pregnancy.

Psoriatic arthritis can be treated with sulphasalazine, steroids or cyclosporine during pregnancy.

Treatment in lactation: Regarding lactating women the first line of treatment is with emollients and low to medium potency corticosteroids. UVB therapy in lactating women is considered to be safe and is indicated as a second-line treatment in these patients. Other drugs as methotrexate, acitretin, cyclosporine and psoralen (PUVA) are contraindicated during breastfeeding.

Biologicals like adalimumab, etanercept and infliximab (anti-TNF-α) and Ustekinumab (IL-12 and 23). The data and experience with these agents is limited for use during pregnancy or breastfeeding.

Topical therapies consisting of emollients and low- to moderate-potency topical steroids constitute first-line therapy for patients with limited psoriasis in pregnancy or lactation. The second-line treatment for pregnant women is narrowband ultraviolet B phototherapy or broadband ultraviolet B, if narrowband ultraviolet B is not available. The tumor necrosis factor-α inhibitors (adalimumab, etanercept, and infliximab) as well as cyclosporine and systemic steroids (in second and third trimesters) may be used with caution in cases unresponsive to above.[9]

TREATMENT OF PSORIASIS IN PREGNANCY

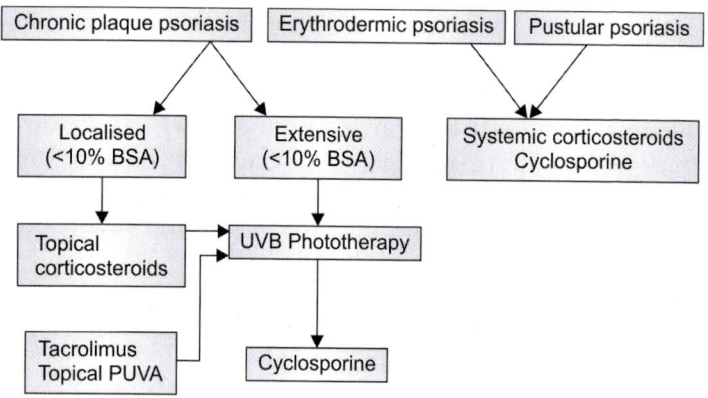

Key Points

- Psoriasis usually improves in pregnancy.
- Such females often have post-partum flare.
- Role of IL-10, altered immune response (Th2 dominance over Th1).
- Pregnancy can precipitate erythrodermic or pustular psoriasis.
- Impetigo Herpeteformis: Form of pustular psoriasis in pregnancy.
- Therapeutic options include topical and systemic corticosteroids, tacrolimus, UVB phototherapy, cyclosporine.

DRUGS USED IN PSORIASIS

Drug	Pregnancy category	Remarks
Corticosteroids	C	Topicals used for limited disease. Systemic used rarely in pustular or erythrodermic psoriasis.
Tacrolimus	C	Preferred in flexures or face
Coal tar	C	Usually not preferred.
Tazarotene	X	Teratogenic.
Anthralin	C	Unacceptable. Not preferred.
Calcipotriol	C	Limited data.
UVB	–	Safe. Used for extensive disease or limited form not responding to topical therapy.
PUVA	C (Psoralen)	Topical can be used in localised cases, e.g. palmoplantar psoariasis. Systemic not used.
Methotrexate	X	Teratogenic. Contraindicated. Avoid pregnancy for 3 months after stopping the drug.
Azathioprine	D	–
Acitretin	X	Teratogenic. Contraindicated. Avoid pregnancy for 3 years after stopping the drug.
Biologicals adalimumab, etanercept, infliximab, ustekinumab.	B	Limited data available for use in pregnancy.

REFERENCES

1. Raychaudhuri SP, Navare T, Gross J, Raychaudhuri SK. Clinical course of psoriasis during pregnancy. Int J Dermatol 2003 Jul;42(7):518–20.

2. Thaxton JE, Sharma S. Interleukin-10: A multi-faceted agent of pregnancy. Am J Reprod Immunol 2010 Jun;63(6):482–91.

3. Patricia Shu Kurizky, Clarissa de Castro Ferreira, Lucas Souza Carmo Nogueira, and Licia Maria Henrique da Mota. Treatment of psoriasis

and psoriatic arthritis during pregnancy and breastfeeding. An Bras Dermatol 2015 May-Jun;90(3):367–75.

4. Yang YW, Chen CS, Chen YH, Lin HC. Psoriasis and pregnancy outcomes: A nationwide population-based study. J Am Acad Dermatol 2011 Jan;64(1):71–7.

5. Lima XT, Janakiraman V, Hughes MD, Kimball AB. The impact of psoriasis on pregnancy outcomes. J Invest Dermatol 2012 Jan;132(1): 85–91.

6. Rogerio Nabor Kondo, Fernanda Mendes Araújo, Allamanda Moura Pereira, Vivian Cristina Holanda Lopes, and Ligia Márcia Mario Martins. Pustular psoriasis of pregnancy (Impetigo herpetiformis)—Case report An Bras Dermatol 2013 Nov-Dec;88(6 Suppl 1):186–9.

7. Ruiz V, Manubens E, Puig L. Psoriasis in pregnancy: A review (I) Actas Dermosifiliogr 2014 Oct;105(8):734–43.

8. Sophie Weatherhead, Stephen C Robson, Nick J Reynolds. Management of psoriasis in pregnancy. BMJ 2007 Jun 9;334(7605): 1218–20.

9. Bae YS, Van Voorhees AS, Hsu S, Korman NJ, Lebwohl MG, Young M, Bebo B Jr, Kimball AB; Review of treatment options for psoriasis in pregnant or lactating women: from the Medical Board of the National Psoriasis Foundation. J Am Acad Dermatol 2012 Sep;67(3):459–77.

7

Nail Psoriasis

Sushil Tahiliani, Harsh Tahiliani

INTRODUCTION

Psoriasis is a chronic inflammatory disease which causes significant distress and morbidity. The etiology is multifactorial and its incidence ranges from 2 to 4% in different populations. The disease may range from mild localized to severe erythrodermic forms.

Nail psoriasis is also known as psoriasis unguis. It was first described by Robert Willan in 1808.

Nail may be involved in up to 50% cases and is often overlooked.[1] Nail psoriasis is associated with psoriatic arthropathy and the incidence (50–86%) in this group is even higher. Psoriasis with nail lesions as the only clinical feature has also been reported. Severe nail psoriasis causes significant functional and social impairment. Nail psoriasis is difficult to treat as compared skin to lesions of psoriasis due to the challenge of delivering therapeutic concentrations of the drugs to various areas of the nail unit.

Clinical Features

The clinical picture of nail psoriasis is varied and depends on the part of the nail apparatus involved along with extent. Psoriasis may involve any part of the nail apparatus. The common nail changes include pitting, onycholysis, subungual hyperkeratosis, nail plate discoloration, uneven nail surface, splinter hemorrhages and paronychia (Table 7.1).[2]

- *Pitting*: Pits are superficial depressions in the nail plate. Pits may be present in normal individuals or in other dermatoses, however, pitting in psoriasis has certain characteristics that

Table 7.1: Diagnostic and non-diagnostic signs of nail psoriasis

Diagnostic	Non-diagnostic
Irregular pitting	Subungual hyperkeratosis
Salmon patches	Splinter hemorrhages
Onycholysis with red border	Nail crumbling
	Paronychia
	Nail plate abnormalities
	Trachyonychia

provide a clue to diagnosis. The proximal matrix is responsible for producing the superficial layer of the nail plate. The presence of parakeratotic cells in the stratum corneum in the proximal matrix cause disruption of normal keratinization. When these foci of parakeratosis are exposed to the environment as the nail grows, they are cast off producing pitting.[3] Finger nails are more commonly affected by pitting. The pits are deep, irregular, small (less than 1 mm in diameter) and randomly arranged in psoriasis. Rarely large, solitary, punched out pits (elkonyxis) producing holes in the nail plate are seen.

- *Leukonychia*: Involvement of ventral and intermediate matrix as compared to dorsal matrix produces leukonychia.

- *Onycholysis and discoloration*: Parakeratosis of the nail bed or hyponychium is responsible for producing focal onycholysis. Nail bed involvement produces areas of red brown discoloration beneath the nail plate. These oily patches are called 'oil spots' or 'salmon patches.' Onycholysis causes entry of air in the space between the nail bed and the nail plate leading to whitish discoloration of the nails. Onycholytic nails are more prone to superinfection with various micro-organisms like yeasts, dermatophytes and bacteria. A red lunula signifies distal matrix involvement.[4]

- *Subungual hyperkeratosis*: Deposition and collection of cells under the nail plate that do not undergo desquamation results in subungual hyperkeratosis. The subungual scales are silver white in color. This sign indicates psoriatic inflammation of the distal nail bed and hyponychium.

- *Splinter hemorrhages*: Psoriatic inflammation in the nail bed dermis produces dilated capillaries which rupture giving rise to splinter hemorrhages. They appear in the distal portion of the nail as thin red or black longitudinal lines. They are usually seen on the fingernails.

- *Crumbling of the nail plate and onychodystrophies*: Beau's lines, ridging and splitting of the nail plate cause onychorrhexis, crumbling of the nail plate and trachyonychia. These changes result from diffuse involvement of the nail apparatus.[4]

- *Paronychia*: Involvement of periungual skin and proximal nail fold causes paronychia. It is commonly seen as an adverse effect of systemic retinoid therapy for psoriasis.[5]

- Pustular psoriasis in the form of Acrodermatitis continua of Hallopeau can affect the nails. Pustules in the nail bed, onycholysis, erythema and pain are the presenting features. Severe cases present with a detached nail plate. The disease is localized to the nail bed and periungual skin.[6]

Nail psoriasis is often believed to be precipitated or worsened by microtrauma due to Koebner phenomenon. The fact that nail psoriasis is more severe in the dominant hand provides evidence for this belief (Table 7.2).

Differential Diagnosis

Nail involvement is present in many inflammatory and infectious diseases. Associated skin lesions provide clues to the diagnosis. Cases with only nail signs are more challenging to diagnose. Psoriasis of toe nails produces only non-diagnostic changes and is more difficult to diagnose. The following diseases should be ruled out:

- *Onychomycosis*: Mycology studies (KOH smear and culture) are mandatory in all cases. However, positive mycology studies do

Table 7.2: Nail changes in psoriasis

Nail area affected	Clinical manifestations
Matrix	Pitting, leukonychia, red lunula
Nail bed	Salmon patches, onycholysis, sub ungual hyperkeratosis
Nail plate	Crumbling of the nail plate
Nail folds	Paronychia

not rule out psoriasis. Pathology of nail clippings and nail bed biopsies may be useful.

- *Alopecia areata*: Pits are small and superficial. They are arranged regularly in a grid-like pattern (scotch plate nails).
- *Eczema*: Nail folds and pulp of the digit are also involved. Differentiating from psoriasis may be difficult in some cases.
- *Lichen planus*: Thinning of the nail plate, ridging, fissuring, pterygium unguis, pulp tent sign suggest towards a diagnosis of lichen planus.
- *Traumatic onycholysis*: Common in toe nails, absence of sugungual hyperkeratosis. May be associated with splinter hemorrhages and subungual hematoma.
- Other conditions like crusted scabies, pityriasis rubra pilaris, parakeratosis pustulosa, inflammatory linear verrucous epidermal nevus and Bazex paraneoplastic acrokeratosis may also mimic psoriasis of nails.

ASSESSMENT OF NAIL PSORIASIS

A. Histopathology

A nail biopsy is sometimes needed to confirm the diagnosis. A biopsy of the nail plate and nail bed is generally done. Hyperkeratosis with hemorrhage in the stratum corneum, hypergranulosis, epidermal hyperplasia, spongiosis and dilated vessels in the dermis are the diagnostic findings.

B. Severity Scores

Evaluation of psoriatic nails by precise measurements of nail thickness, optical profilometry of the depth and area of pits has been done. These methods are complicated. Nail psoriasis severity index (NAPSI) is an easy, reproducible and comprehensive method to evaluate the extent of nail disease.[7]

- The nail is divided into 4 quadrants.
- Each nail is graded (0–4) for matrix involvement. Pitting, leukonychia, red lunula and crumbling of nail plate signify matrix disease.
- Each nail is graded (0–4) for nail bed disease. Salmon patches, onycholysis, subungual hyperkeratosis and splinter hemorr-hages signify nail bed disease.

- Absence of signs is graded as 0, 1 if present in 1 quadrant, 2 if present in 2 quadrants, 3 if present in 3 quadrants and 4 if all quadrants are involved.
- The sum of nail matrix and nail bed disease (0–8) is done for each nail. 10 nail NAPSI (out of 80) or 20 nail NAPSI (out of 160) can be calculated.
- If a target score is desired, all 8 parameters can be judged individually in each quadrant giving that nail a score of 0–32.

NAPSI evaluated along with dermatological life quality index correlates better with severity of disease as compared to only one method. These scores in conjunction are used to evaluate severity as well as therapeutic responses.

Treatment

Nail psoriasis is refractory and requires long periods of treatment. Spontaneous improvement is known to occur in a few cases. Many newer treatment options are available for skin lesions of psoriasis, however, the options for nail psoriasis have poor efficacy and treatment compliance.

A. Topical Therapies

- Superpotent topical corticosteroids over the proximal nail fold under occlusion are effective for nail matrix disease.[8,9] For nail bed disease the nail plate should be trimmed to the hyponychium and the steroid applied as close to the nail bed as possible. Topical corticosteroids can be combined with salicylic acid.
- A comparative study by Tosti et al proved twice daily application of calcipotriol ointment to be as effective as high potency steroids.[10] Concurrent treatment with vitamin D_3 analogues and topical corticosteroids is more efficacious than either agent used alone.[11] However, both agents have their own side effects on long-term use.
- Tazarotene gel applied with or without occlusion for 24 weeks is effective for all types of nail psoriasis.[12]
- One percent topical 5-FU, topical cyclosporine in an oily preparation and short contact anthralin (0.4–2%) therapy have shown some improvement in isolated cases.

B. Intralesional Therapy

- Triamcinolone acetonide (2.5–10 mg/ml) injected into the proximal nail fold for matrix disease and into the nail bed through the hyponychium or lateral nail fold for nail bed disease is effective.[13] The injections should be repeated every 3–4 weeks. Intralesional injections for nail psoriasis are extremely painful and the skin must be cooled before injecting to reduce the pain or local anesthesia given.

C. Radiation Therapy

- PUVA (topical as well as oral) has caused remission of nail psoriasis in various studies. It had better results in clearing nail bed disease as compared to matrix involvement but contradictory reports of worsening of nail psoriasis due to PUVA also exist.

- There exists variable evidence for superficial radiotherapy, grenz rays and electron beam therapy in nail psoriasis, however, all forms of radiation have potential serious side effects and their use is limited in the clinical setting.

D. Systemic Therapy

Systemic therapy is indicated when nail psoriasis is associated with severe cutaneous disease or arthropathy. It should also be considered in patients with only nail disease that causes significant functional and psychosocial morbidity.

- Low dose acitretin therapy (0.2–0.3 mg/kg/day) improves matrix as well as nail bed disease. Doses higher than 0.3 mg/kg/day lead to thinning of normal nails, paronychia and periungual pyogenic granulomas.[5]

- Cyclosporine 3 mg/kg/day[14] was effective in improving nail disease in a 10-week trial. Methotrexate, azathiprine, mycophenolate mofetil and hydroxyurea have been used in individual cases but there is a lack of documented data demonstrating their efficacy.

- Biologics like infliximab,[15] adalimumab, etanercept have caused remission and improvement in nail psoriasis. Secukinumab[16] has shown promising results in phase II trials.

E. Combination Therapy

Use of rational combinations of more than one treatment modality targets more than one pathway of pathogenesis and better results can be obtained.

F. Surgery

Avulsion of the nails by chemical (urea ointment) or surgical means may be needed for painful, refractory and distorted nails. Elective ablation of the matrix during surgery prevents regrowth of the diseased nail.

REFERENCES

1. Crawford GM. Psoriasis of the nails. Arch Derm Syphilol 1938;38: 583–94.
2. Dawber RPR, Baran R, de Berker D. Disorders of Nails. In: Textbook of Dermatology. 6th edn. Hoboken, New Jersey: Blackwell Science; 1998, p. 2815–68.
3. Zaias N. The nail in health and disease, 2nd ed. Norwalk: Appleton and Lange; 1990.
4. Baran R, Dawber RPR. The nail in dermatological diseases. In: Baran R, Dawber RPR, editors. Diseases of the nails and their management. 2nd ed. Oxford: Blackwell Scientific Publications, 1994, p. 135–73.
5. Baran R. Retinoids and the nails. J Dermatol Treat 1990;1:151–4.
6. Piraccini BM, Tosti A, Lorizzo M, et al. Pustular psoriasis of the nails. Treatment and long-term follow-up of 46 patients. Br J Dermatol 2001;144:1000–5.
7. Rich P, Scher RK. Nail psoriasis severity index: A useful tool for evaluation of nail psoriasis. J Am Acad Dermatol 2003;49:206–12.
8. Jiaravuthisan MM, Sasseville D, Vendor RB, et al. Psoriasis of the nail: anatomy, pathology, clinical presentation and a review of literature on therapy. J Am Acad Dermatol 2007;57:1–27.
9. de Berker DAR. Management of nail psoriasis. Clin Exp Dermatol 2000; 25:357–62.
10. Tosti A, Piraccini BM, Cameli N, Kokely F, Plozzer C, Cannata GE, et al. Calcipotriol ointment in nail psoriasis; a controlled double-blind comparision with betamethasone dipropionate and salicylic acid. Br J Dermatol 1998;139:655–9.
11. Rigopoulos D, Ioannides D, Prastitis N, Katsambas A. Nail psoriasis: A combined treatment using calcipotriol cream and clobetasol propionate cream. Acta Derm Venereol 2002;82:140.

12. Scher RK, Stiller M, Zhu YI. Tazarotene 0.1% gel in the treatment of fingernail psoriasis: a double-blind, randomized, vehicle-controlled study. Cutis 2001;68:355–8.

13. de Berker DAR, Lawrence CM. A simplified protocol of steroid injection for psoriatic nail dystrophy. Br J Dermatol 1998;138:90–5.

14. Mahrle G, Schulze HJ, Farber L, et al. Low-dose short-term cyclosporine versus etretinate in psoriasis; Improvement of skin, nail and joint involvement. J Am Acad Dermatol 1995;32:78–88.

15. Reich K, Nestle FO, Papp K, et al. Infliximab induction and maintenance therapy for moderate to severe psoriasis: A phase III, multicentre, double-blind trial: Lancet 2005;366:1367–74.

16. Paul C, Reich K, Gottlieb AB, Mrowietz U, Philipp S, Nakayama J, Harfst E, Guettner A, Papavassilis C; CAIN457A2211 study group. Secukinumab improves hand, foot and nail lesions in moderate-to-severe plaque psoriasis: Subanalysis of a randomized, double-blind, placebo-controlled, regimen-finding phase 2 trial. J Eur Acad Dermatol Venereol 2014;28(12):1670–5.

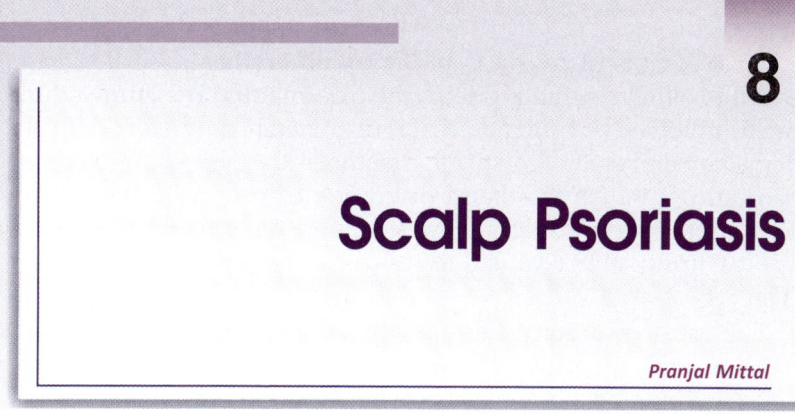

8

Scalp Psoriasis

Pranjal Mittal

INTRODUCTION

Scalp is a well-known predilection site for psoriasis.[1]

Scalp psoriasis around the hairline, can cause significant impairment in quality of life due to its visibility.

Around 50% to 80% patients, present with scalp involvement alone or in conjunction with lesions in other areas.[2]

The scalp, together with the face, is one of the parts most affected by psoriasis in childhood and adolescence.

The clinical presentation of scalp psoriasis can be varied, ranging from mild to extremely severe. The lesions can involve the hairline and extend beyond, affecting the facial area, with visible desquamation and plaques.

Scalp psoriasis is difficult to treat, due to the inaccessible nature of the scalp and its proximity to the facial area.[3]

The choice of an appropriate vehicle is crucial to increase patient compliance. While scalp psoriasis can often be treated adequately with topical therapy, recalcitrant disease may require more aggressive approaches, including systemic agents.

CLINICAL PRESENTATION

Scalp psoriasis is often the first manifestation of the disease. It may be sustained for years despite remission in other areas. It may be associated with different types of psoriasis: Psoriasis vulgaris, chronic plaque psoriasis, guttate psoriasis, inverse psoriasis, pustular psoriasis, erythrodermic psoriasis, psoriatic arthritis or nail psoriasis.

Scalp lesions of psoriasis present with erythema, scaling and pruritus, often resembling seborrheic dermatitis. The entire scalp can be involved but other times it is restricted to only a few sharply demarcated plaques. A distinctive feature is the presence of "corona psoriatica", which is a band or corona of psoriasis, projecting beyond the hairline on the forehead. Uncommonly, the scales may appear firmly adherent and asbestos-like (pityriasis amiantacea) (Fig. 8.1).

The most common locations are behind the ears, above the hairline, and in peripheral areas of the face, such as the temples and the upper part of the back of the neck (Fig. 8.2).

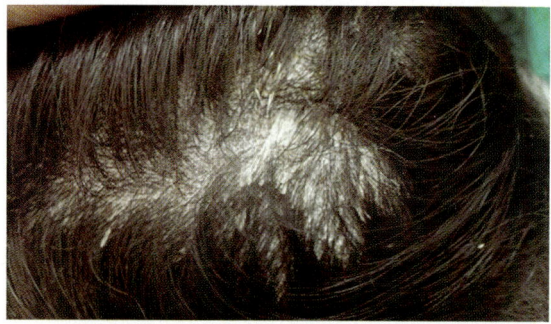

Fig. 8.1 Thick "asbestos-like" scales (pityriasis amiantacea)

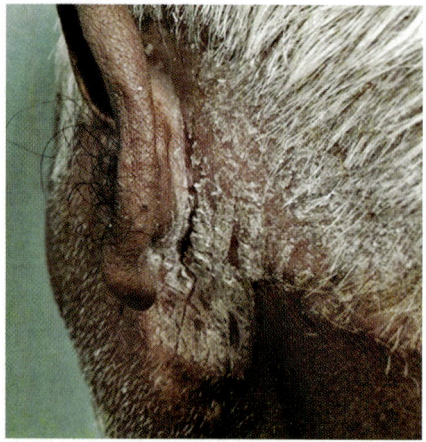

Fig. 8.2 Patient with scalp psoriasis. Involvement of the skin beyond the hairline, extending behind the ear, in the form of visible, well-defined, silver-white, scaly plaques

The most common symptoms of concern are desquamation and pruritus.[4]

Hairloss is not a feature of scalp psoriasis, although telogen effluvium and reduction of hair density may occur in the areas of the plaques. In a few extensive lesions in erythrodermic forms, cases of scarring alopecia have been reported.[2]

DIFFERENTIAL DIAGNOSIS

Scalp involvement strongly suggests the possibility of psoriasis and thus, the commonly affected areas, such as the knees, elbows and nails should be inspected for psoriatic lesions.

- Psoriasis may coexist with seborrheic dermatitis and these two conditions may be histologically indistinguishable. The scales in seborrheic dermatitis are greasy and lesions rarely extend beyond the hairline, whereas in psoriasis, the scales are dry and lesions extend beyond the hairline. Unless there is complete confluence, the individual lesions are discrete, in contrast to seborrheic dermatitis, which is less well defined. Psoriasis may develop from seborrheic dermatitis with a Koebner response secondary to colonization by Malassezia yeast. This has been described as *sebopsoriasis*.[5]
- Lichen simplex chronicus in the occipital area, can be differentiated by being very pruritic.
- Tinea amiantacea is characterized by thick, "asbestos-like" scaling of the scalp and temporary alopecia. Whereas hairloss is not a feature of scalp psoriasis.

The other differentials are mentioned in Table 8.1.

Table 8.1: Differential diagnosis of scalp psoriasis

Seborrheic dermatitis

Lichen simplex chronicus (occipital area)

Atopic dermatitis with superinfection

Pityriasis rubra pilaris

Cutaneous mycosis (tinea capitis, etc.)

Subacute lupus erythematosus

Dermatomyositis with scalp involvement

Bowen's disease (isolated plaques)

Pemphigus foliaceous

EFFECT ON QUALITY OF LIFE

The chronic nature of scalp psoriasis may have a major psychological impact on sufferers, even though it is not a life-threatening disease. Moderate to severe forms of scalp psoriasis have been shown to impose considerable limitations on quality of life in aspects such as vacations, work, interpersonal relations, sexual relations.

Psoriasis Disability Index (PDI) and Scalpdex are useful and reproducible tools, developed in recent years, to evaluate quality of life.

Scalpdex is an instrument, which investigates and evaluates the available treatments to detect therapeutic benefits to the quality of life of patients, by intrapersonal and interpersonal comparisons.[6]

The index comprising of 23 items, has been specifically developed to measure quality of life in individuals with scalp dermatitis.[7]

THERAPEUTIC APPROACH

Treatment should be tailored to each individual in order to achieve a good clinical response, which lasts for as long as possible.[8]

This form of psoriasis is more difficult to treat than the common form affecting the rest of the body, due to scalp inaccessibility and greater thickness of the plaques.

The different therapeutic options available for scalp psoriasis have been discussed here.

A. Topical therapeutic agents

Topical treatment forms the therapeutic basis for scalp psoriasis.

Most commonly used treatments for scalp psoriasis include:
- Keratolytic agents (salicylic acid in concentrations higher than 2%, urea at concentrations of between 10% and 40%, alpha hydroxy acids, glycolic acid, resorcin)
- Coal tar
- Dithranol (anthralin)
- Antifungals (1.5% ciclopiroxolamine, 2% ketoconazole, 2% clotrimazole)
- Retinoids (tazarotene)
- Corticosteroids (medium or high potency)
- Vitamin D analogues
  - Calcitriol

- Tacalcitol
- Calcipotriol

Most commonly used vehicles are: acceptance by patient (higher to lower)

- Shampoo
- Alcohol-based lotions
- Gels
- Foams
- Emulsions
- Creams
- Ointments

Sequential therapeutic strategy in the topical treatment of scalp psoriasis according to the review by Koo et al[9] (Table 8.2).

Table 8.2: Sequential therapeutic strategy

Treatment phase	Active ingredients
Clearing (2 weeks)	Clobetasol or betamethasone propionate + calcipotriol (twice daily for 2 weeks)
Transition (2 weeks)	Clobetasol or betamethasone propionate on weekends + calcipotriol during the week (twice daily for 2 weeks)
Maintenance (long term)	Long-term calcipotriol

B. Phototherapy

It has been one of the most traditional treatments for psoriasis. It is currently reserved for lesions resistant to topical treatment.

Systemic psoralen plus UVA (PUVA) treatment, narrowband (311 nm) UVB therapy, topical PUVA, and other varieties, such as 308 nm excimer laser or microphototherapy, may be used.

Systemic PUVA treatment is being displaced by narrowband UVB treatment, with a regimen of 3 sessions per week. It is more convenient as the patient do not have to take psoralen or use sunglasses to protect themselves from sunlight.[8]

C. Grenz Rays

Grenz rays use electromagnetic radiation, with less penetration. Its use with betamethasone propionate have shown to clear up lesions more faster with longer remissions.[10]

D. Systemic Treatment

Systemic treatment is considered when patients do not respond to topical treatment or when lesions occur on other areas of the body. There is no difference between the different classic systemic treatments, such as methotrexate, cyclosporine, acitretin, or fumaric acid salts, and current biologic treatments, such as efalizumab, etanercept, infliximab, and adalimumab, for the treatment of scalp psoriasis.

TREATMENT ALGORITHM

Figure 8.3 presents the treatment algorithm for severe scalp psoriasis.[11]

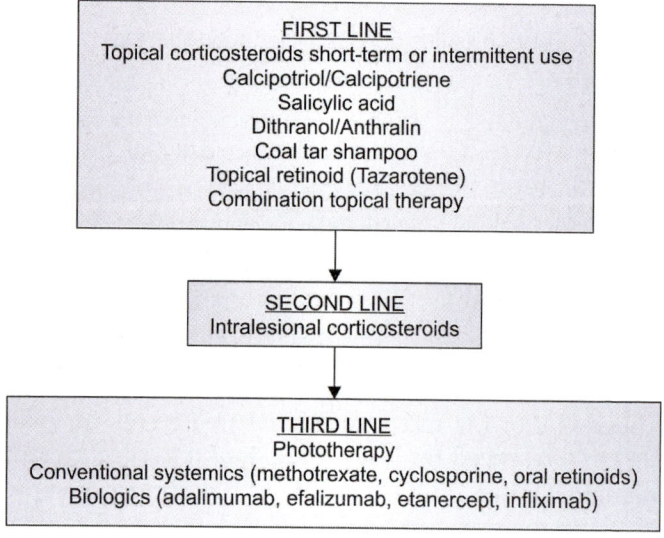

Fig. 8.3 Treatment algorithm

REFERENCES

1. Raychaudhuri SP, Gross J. A comparative study of pediatric onset psoriasis with adult onset psoriasis. Pediatr Dermatol 2000;17(3): 174–8.
2. Papp K, Berth-Jones J, Kragballe K, de la Brasinne M. Scalp psoriasis: A review of current topical treatment options. JEADV 2007;21: 1151–60.
3. Sola-Ortigosa J, Sanchez-Regana M, Umbert-Millet P. An update on scalp psoriasis. Actas Dermosifiliogr 2009 Sep;100(7):536–43.

4. Van der Kerkhof, de Hoop D, de Korte J, Kuipers MV. Scalp psoriasis, clinical presentations and therapeutic management. J Dermatol. 1998;197:326–34.

5. Gupta AK, Batra R, Bluhm R, Boekhout T, Dawson TL Jr. Skin diseases associated with Malassezia species. J Am Acad Dermatol 2004;51: 785–98.

6. Vanaclocha F, Puig L, Daudén E, Escudero J, Hernanz JM, Ferrándiz C, et al. Validación de la versiónespañola del cuestionario Psoriasis Disability Index en la evaluación de la calidad de vidaenpacientes con psoriasis moderada-grave. Actas Dermosifiliogr 2005;96:659–68.

7. Chen SC, Yeung J, Vhren M-M. Scalpdex: A quality of life instrument for scalp dermatitis. Arch Dermatol 2002;138:803–7.

8. Sánchez-Regaña M, Umbert P. Actualizaciónen eltratamiento de la psoriasis. Dermatología Práctica 2008;16:5–16.

9. Koo J, Blum R, Lebwohl M. A randomized, multicentre study of calcipotriene ointment and clobetasol propionatefoam in the sequential treatment of localized plaque-type psoriasis: short-and long-term outcomes. J Am Acad Dermatol 2006;55:637–41.

10. Johannesson A, Lindelof B. Additional effect of Grenz rays on psoriasis lesions of the scalp treated with topical corticosteroids. Dermatologica 1987;175:290–2.

11. Chan CS, Van Voorhees AS, Lebwohl MG, Korman NJ, Young M, Bebo BF Jr, Kalb RE, Hsu S. Treatment of severe scalp psoriasis: From the Medical Board of the National Psoriasis Foundation. J Am Acad Dermatol 2009 Jun;60(6):962–71.

9

Psoriasis and Comorbidities

Sunanda Mahajan

INTRODUCTION

Psoriasis is an immunologically mediated chronic inflammatory disease in genetically predisposed individuals affecting approximately 1–3% of the general population. Comorbidity is the presence of one or more additional disorders (or diseases) co-occurring with a primary disease or disorder; or the effect of such additional disorders or diseases. Psoriasis is found to be, associated with significant comorbidity (Table 9.1), for example, metabolic syndrome (MS) and coronary heart disease (CHD). These co-morbidities are likely linked to underlying chronic inflammatory nature of psoriasis. Thus commonly seen in moderate to severe psoriasis.

Comorbidities may increase with age. Psoriatic patients had a 4-fold increased risk of type 2 diabetes, 3-fold risk of myocardial infarction and life expectancy shortened by 4 years compared to healthy controls.

Factors that may contribute to comorbidities in psoriasis

Environmental risk factors: Smoking and obesity, stress, drugs

- *Genes and loci associated with psoriasis, diabetes, and cardiovascular disease*: PSORS2/3/4, CDKAL1, ApoE4, and TNFAIP3.
- *Mediating factors*: Pathophysiology,
  TH1/17 inflammation (atherosclerosis, thrombosis, lipid metabolism)
- Epidermal proliferation—(uric acid, oxidative stress)
  Angiogenesis—(endothelial dysfunction)

Table 9.1: Classification of comorbidities associated with psoriasis

Classic	Psoriatic arthritis
	Inflammatory bowel disease
	Psychological and psychiatric disorders
	Uveitis
Emerging	Metabolic syndrome and its components
	Cardiovascular diseases
	Atherosclerosis
	Nonalcoholic fatty liver disease
	Lymphomas
	Sleep apnea
	Chronic obstructive pulmonary disease
	Osteoporosis
	Parkinson's disease
	Celiac disease
	Erectile dysfunction
Related to lifestyle	Smoking habit
	Alcoholism
	Anxiety
Related to treatment	Dyslipidemia (acitretin and cyclosporine)
	Nephrotoxicity (cyclosporine)
	Hypertension (cyclosporine)
	Hepatotoxicity (methotrexate, leflunomide and acitretin)
	Skin cancer (PUVA)

- Treatment
  - s Increase CV risk—(e.g. cyclosporine, acitretin)
  - s Decrease CV risk—(e.g. methotrexate)
- *Psychosocial impact of psoriasis:* Depression, alcohol and smoking, lower socioeconomic status.

Psoriasis involves a complex interplay between various cells of the immune system and skin, including dermal dendritic cells, T cells, neutrophils and keratinocytes.

Sustained skin inflammation is sufficient to induce secretion of cytokines from subcutaneous fat cells, endothelial cells and other inflammatory cells, leading to endothelial dysfunction, vascular inflammation, and systemic inflammation. Systemic inflammation in turn causes insulin resistance, a state in which the equilibrium between proatherogenic and antiatherogenic effects of insulin is shifted towards proatherogenic effects. This shift expedites endothelial dysfunction, which then leads to atherosclerosis and eventually myocardial infarction if coronary arteries are involved.

'Psoriatic march' is a recently defined term and has been used to describe this process developing in a stepwise manner. These psoriatic cytokines can favor the development of psoriatic arthritis (PsA), and mediate a number of metabolic effects that may lead to progression of insulin resistance, dyslipidemia and non-alcoholic fatty liver disease (NAFLD), hence directly and/or indirectly favoring the development of atherosclerosis.

An early and effective psoriasis treatment could be effective in blocking the progression of the psoriatic march by controlling the skin inflammation and thus preventing the natural progression. On the other hand, it is also possible to hypothesize that metabolic comorbidities such as obesity, NAFLD and metabolic syndrome might actively contribute to the severity of psoriasis through the release of pathogenetic mediators from the inflamed liver and/or visceral adipose tissues, including increased reactive oxygen species, elevated C reactive protein (CRP), IL-6 and adipokines, which also interfere with thrombosis.

OBESITY AND METABOLIC SYNDROME

A strong association between obesity, increased body mass index (BMI) and psoriasis has been found. The risk of obesity increased with the severity of psoriasis and was higher for patients with a longer psoriasis history.

Common cytokine pathways are responsible for both psoriasis and obesity but it is yet to be answered which pathology comes first when psoriasis-associated obesity and the metabolic syndrome is considered.

Both psoriasis and obesity are chronic inflammatory states. Intra-abdominal fat acts like an endocrine organ, secreting pro-inflammatory cytokines (adipocytokines) (Fig. 9.1)—under the influence of inflammatory mediators such as TNF-α that is produced by the skin, promoting inflammation, primary cytokines that are produced by adipocytes include IL-6, TNF-α, plasminogen activator inhibitor type 1 (PAI-1), leptin and adiponectin, each of which plays multiple roles in inflammation, glucose metabolism and endothelial cell function.

As systemic inflammation continues and with increasing BMI, adiponectin is downregulated while leptin and resistin are

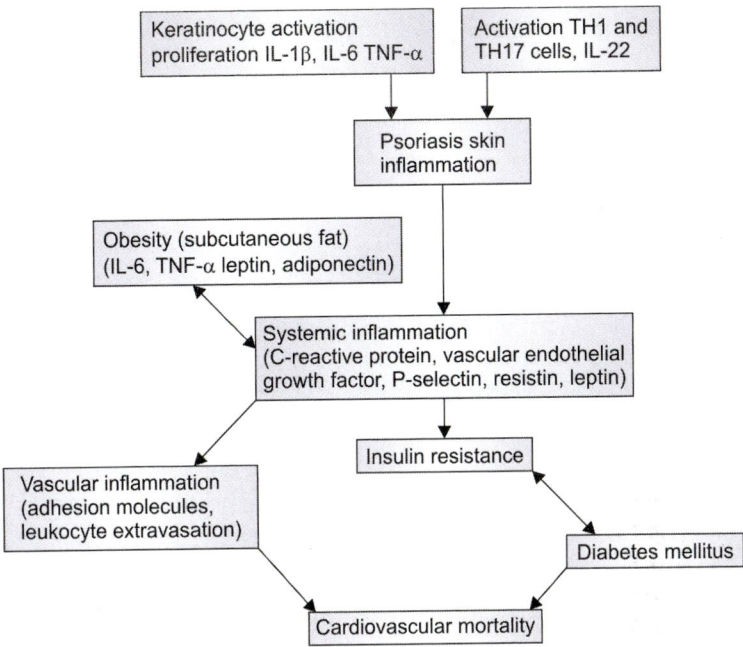

Fig. 9.1 Simplified mechanism of systemic inflammation and consequent events

upregulated, which induces insulin resistance and causes endothelial cells to produce adhesion molecules, promoting a hepatic release of both fibrinogen and C-reactive protein, and augmenting the procoagulant effects on platelets. These drive the process with consequences of metabolic syndrome.

Besides, adipocytes bear toll-like receptors that behave as a component of innate immunity and allow an immediate response to foreign pathogens and release cytokines.

Patients with a greater BMI were found to have a lower likelihood of achieving significant clinical improvement of their psoriasis despite receiving equivalent doses of the medication. Treatment with cyclosporine also has been proven to be more efficacious when coupled with a low-calorie diet and moderate weight loss (Table 9.2).

MANAGEMENT

Psoriasis, with its comorbidities, must be approached in a multidisciplinary manner to effectively and comprehensively

Table 9.2: The new International Diabetes Federation (IDF) definition

According to the new IDF definition, for persons to be defined as having the metabolic syndrome they must have:
Central obesity (defined as waist circumference* with ethnicity specific values)
Plus any two of the following four factors:

Raised triglycerides	≥150 mg/dL (1.7 mmol/L) or specific treatment for this lipid abnormality
Reduced HDL cholesterol	<40 mg/dL (1.03 mmol/L) in males <50 mg/dL (1.29 mmol/L) in females or specific treatment for this lipid abnormality
Raised blood pressure	Systolic BP ≥ or diastolic BP ≥85 mm Hg or treatment of previously diagnosed hypertension
Raised fasting plasma glucose	(FPG) ≥100 mg/dL (5.6 mmol/L) or previously diagnosed type 2 diabetes If above 5.6 mmol/L or 100 mg/dL, OGTT is strongly recommended but is not necessary to define presence of the syndrome.

if BMI is >30 kg/m², central obesity can be assumed and waist circumference does not need to be measured.

understand, manage, and treat those with this complex disorder:

- First, a diagnosis of psoriasis should trigger a high clinical suspicion and investigation for a potential coexistence of the metabolic syndrome, cardiovascular risk factors and comorbidities
- Checklist to detect comorbidities (Table 9.3) and lifestyle factors (e.g. smoking habits and alcoholism); application of scales to assess anxiety and depression, questioning about sexual dysfunction during history-taking.
- Clinical examination (body weight, height, BMI, waist circumference) and an ophthalmologic examination.
- Assess the severity of psoriasis (PASI and DLQI); and to request laboratory tests (blood glucose, lipidogram, liver profile and renal function).
- Counsel patients—need for lifestyle modification—smoking cessation, weight reduction and regular screening for diabetes and hypertension.

Table 9.3: Important comorbidities and screening recommendations

Comorbidity	Suggested screening
Diabetes mellitus	Fasting blood glucose
Arterial hypertension	Two consecutive blood pressure measurements
Obesity	Body mass index
	Waist circumference
Dyslipidemia	Fasting blood lipids
Cardiovascular disease	Screening for the components of the metabolic syndrome
Liver disease	Transaminases[†]
Psoriatic arthritis	Screening questionnaire (e.g. ToPAS, PASE, PEST)
	Ask/look for tender/swollen joints
	Ask for inflammatory back pain

ToPAS=Toronto psoriatic arthritis screening; PASE=psoriatic arthritis screening and evaluation; PEST=psoriasis epidemiology screening tool; Coronary artery disease; Recommendations for dermatologists (recommendations in the respective guidelines may vary); [†]Nonalcoholic fatty liver disease (NAFLD) cannot be ruled out on the basis of laboratory tests alone; Typically at night, eases with physical activity

- Therapeutic decision should be discussed with the patient, taking into account his/her comorbidities and lifestyle. Comorbidity necessitates co-medication. Many of these concomitant medications are known to trigger psoriasis.
- Individualized drug therapy—depending on severity and type of psoriasis and taking into consideration the associated comorbidities.
- Non-pharmacological intervention such as diet, smoking cessation, and physical exercise could both improve the response to treatments for psoriasis and reduce the cardiovascular risk.

Early identification and treatment of these comorbid conditions can possibly reduce the morbidity, mortality, and economic burden associated with the disease.

RECOMMENDED READING

1. Armstrong AW, et al. Psoriasis and the risk of diabetes mellitus: a systematic review and meta-analysis. JAMA Dermatol 2013;149:84–91.
2. Augustin M, Glaeske G, Radtke MA, Christophers E, Reich K, Schäfer I. Epidemiology. and comorbidity of psoriasis in children. Br J Dermatol 2010;162:633–6.

3. Cassano N, Vestita M, Apruzzi D, Vena GA. Alcohol, psoriasis, liver disease, and anti-psoriasis drugs. Int J Dermatol 2011;50:1323.

4. Chiang YY, Lin HW. Association between psoriasis and chronic obstructive pulmonary disease: a population-based study in Taiwan. J Eur Acad Dermatol Venereol 2012;26(1):59–65.

5. Christophers E. Comorbidities in psoriasis. J Eur Acad Dermatol Venerol 2006;20:52–5.

6. Cohen AD, et al. Psoriasis and diabetes: A population-based cross sectional study. J Eur Acad Dermatol Venereol 2008;22:585–9.

7. Dreiher J, et al. Psoriasis and chronic obstructive pulmonary disease: A case-control study. Br J Dermatol 2008;159(4):956–60.

8. E. Daudén, et al. Integrated Approach to Comorbidity in Patients With Psoriasis Actas Dermosifiliogr 2012; 103(Supl 1):1–64.

9. Fernandez-Torres RM, Paradela S, Fonseca E. Psoriasis in patients older than 65 years. A comparative study with younger adult psoriatic patients. J Nutr Health Aging 2012;16:586–91.

10. Gelfand JM, Troxel AB, Lewis JD, et al. The risk of mortality in patients with psoriasis: results from a population-based study. Arch Dermatol 2007;143:1493–9.

11. Gelfand JM, Weinstein R, Porter SB, Neimann AL, Berlin JA, Margolis DJ. Prevalence and treatment of psoriasis in the United Kingdom: a population-based study. Arch Dermatol 2005;141:1537–41.

12. Gudjonsson JE, Elder J. Psoriasis. In Fitzpatrick's Dermatology in General Medicine. 7th edn. Wolff K, Goldsmith LA, Katz SI, Gilchrest BA, Paller AS, Leffell DJ (Eds). New York, McGraw-Hill, 2008:169.

13. Karaca S, et al. Might psoriasis be a risk factor for obstructive sleep apnea syndrome. Sleep Breath 2013;17(1):275–80.

14. Kim N, Thrash B, Menter A. Comorbidities in Psoriasis Patients. Semin Cutan Med Surg 2010;29:10–15.

15. Kimball AB, Jacobson C, Weiss S, Vreeland MG, Wu Y. The psycho-social burden of psoriasis. Am J Clin Dermatol 2005;6:383–92.

16. Kurd SK, Gelfand JM. The prevalence of previously diagnosed and undiagnosed psoriasis in US adults: results from NHANES 2003–2004. J Am Acad Dermatol 2009;60:218–24.

17. Nair RP, Henseler T, Jenisch S, et al. Evidence for two psoriasis suscep-tibility loci (HLA and 17q) and two novel candidate regions (16q and 20p) by genome-wide scan. Hum Mol Genet 1997;6:1349–56.

18. Oliveira MFSP, Rocha BO, Duerte GV. Continuing Medical Education—Psoriasis: classical and emerging comorbidities An. Bras. Dermatol 2015;90(1):9–20.

19. Onumah N, Kircik LH. Psoriasis and its comorbidities. J Drugs Dermatol 2012;11:s5–10.

10

Psoriatic Arthritis

Nina Madnani, Kaleem Khan

INTRODUCTION

Psoriatic arthritis (PsA) is a sero-negative debilitating arthritis, often missed in patients of psoriasis. It is characterized by enthesitis, dactylitis, peripheral arthritis and spondylitis. Extra-articular manifestations have been identified, and are regarded as important to the disease evaluation as the joints involved themselves. Delayed diagnosis results in irreversible damage and hence timely recognition is essential.

Incidence

Incidence of PsA in Indian patients with psoriasis is 8.7%,[1] and between 7 and 48% in the western population.[2] Approximately 10 to 20% of patients with PsA will have no skin lesions.

Genetics

The need to search for newer genetic loci for PsA arthritis arise from the important observation that the pattern of inheritance is stronger in patients with PsA than with psoriasis, suggesting more distinct loci encoding for PsA. Although it is difficult to identify the exact inheritance pattern of PsA, certain studies indicate HLA-B27, MHC region. Non-HLA risk loci at IL23R, PTPN22 and Chromosome 5q31 have also been reported.[3] Fitzgerald and colleagues have demonstrated that there is distinct genetic heterogenecity between psoriasis vulgaris and PsA. Furthermore, they have shown that there are different alleles and haplotypes encoding for PsA which can explain the diverse clinical manifestation seen PsA.[4]

Clinical Variants

Five clinical variants have been described.

- Asymmetric oligoarthritis
- Distal interphalangeal
- Symmetric polyarthritis
- Spondylitis with or without sacroiliitis
- Arthritis mutilans

Most frequently reported joint involvement from the Indian subcontinent is the small joints of the hands and feet, followed by sacroiliitis, and lastly the knees.[5] This is in contrast to other countries where sacroiliitis or oligoarthritis may be the commonest presenting feature. The involved joints show signs of enthesitis, which is spontaneous pain and tenderness at the site of tendon insertion. The commonest site is the Achilles tendon insertion. Dactylitis is another characteristic feature of PsA and this presents as spontaneous swelling and redness which may be accompanied with pain. Spondylitis is usually accompanied with peripheral joint disease.

Psoriasis and PsA may not begin concurrently. Psoriasis precedes arthritis in 60–80% of patients. Arthritis precedes psoriasis in 15–20% of patients.

Extra-articular Manifestations

Extra-articular manifestations in PsA are more commonly seen in male patients with axial pattern of joint involvement. PsA is more severe in patients with extra-articular manifestations and the reverse is also true. Smokers are at a significantly higher risk for developing extra-articular changes than non-smokers. Synovitis commonly affects the flexor tendon sheaths, with sparing of the extensor tendon sheath. Subcutaneous nodules are rare.

The commonest organ systems involved include bowel (33.16%) and ocular systems (32.63%) in the form of inflammatory bowel disease and anterior uveitis respectively.[6]

A recent association has been made with the rare phenomenon of peripheral corneal melting syndrome and PsA.[7]

Up to 80% of patients with PsA have associated nail changes, with a wide variation in presentation.[8] Over the years, we have come to recognize the positive co-relation between nail involvement in psoriasis and development of PsA.[9] The paradigm shift in our understanding of nail changes predicting PsA comes from better understanding the anatomy due to direct visualization with newer imaging modalities like ultrasound and MRI.[10] Fibers from the extensor tendon of the DIP joint interdigitate and engulf the nail root while the collateral ligaments merge with the lateral borders of the nail thus proving the intimate relation of the nail with the DIP joints. Enthesitis, which is the hallmark of PsA, will extend into the nail root which in turn may present clinically as changes in the nail.[11]

Investigations

The purpose of investigating the patient is for evaluating disease activity and joint inflammation/destruction, and baseline investigations as a preparation for systemic therapy.

A complete body profile which includes CBC, ESR, LFT and RFT, ANA.

Measurements like BMI, a waist-to-hip ratio for checking central obesity

- RA factor
- ANA
- HLA-B27 status

For biologics to be initiated, ruling out infections both bacterial and viral, is necessary. This includes a battery of tests. A recent evaluation, however, found a little evidence in doing so. The only, strongly recommended, investigation was that for tuberculosis screening. The preferred method was the interferon-gamma release assay test as opposed to the tuberculin skin test.[12]

Biomarkers (soluble proteins and microbiomics) are being actively researched to predict disease progression and therapeutic response. But they have yet to be validated for use in clinical practice.[13]

Radiological Evaluation Should Include

Conventional radiograph of the hands including wrists, when suspecting peripheral disease. The characteristic findings are changes due to bone destruction and proliferation. Classically, the disease changes are asymmetrical with one joint showing more inflammatory/destructive changes than other. Severe bone destruction, as seen in long standing untreated disease or the mutilating variety of disease, presents with narrowing of the heads of metacarpals and metatarsals (penciling). Destruction of the central portion of the articular surface gives the "pencil-in-cup" appearance.

Conventional radiograph of the Sacroiliac (SI) joints when suspecting axial joint involvement.

MRI of the SI joints should be done when conventional radiograph fails to identify axial disease and a strong clinical suspicion remains. It helps to evaluate both active inflammatory lesions and structural lesions.

Ultrasonography is useful not only in detection of peripheral joint involvement but also can pick up subclinical enthesiopathy, degenerative tendinitis, and peri-tendinitis and bursitis. The Achilles tendon is a good site for evaluation in symptomatic patients.[14]

High-frequency ultrasound (linear arrays at 30–35 MHz) imaging of fingers can reliably pick up findings strongly suggestive of PsA. These findings include tenosynovitis, soft tissue inflammation and enthesitis.[15] High-frequency ultrasound also has a prognostic value by quantifying change in inflammation, plaque thickness, synovitis and bone lesions before starting treatment and after variable periods into the treatment schedule.

Power Doppler (PD) has been used to pick up early, subclinical, enthesitis.[16]

Narvaez et al showed that MRI of the hand and wrist in early stages of PsA can easily and definitely help to distinguish PsA from rheumatoid arthritis. The characteristic features include presence of enthesitis and/or extensive diaphyseal bone marrow edema while a strongly suggestive feature was diffuse soft-tissue edema extending into the subcutis.[17] A PsA MRI score (PsAMRIS) has been developed and is currently being evaluated for disease evaluation on MRI with promising results.[18]

Differential Diagnosis

- For polyarticular disease, the closest differential diagnosis is rheumatoid arthritis. A positive RA test, symmetrical, PIP joint involvement without enthesitis points to a diagnosis of rheumatoid arthritis. Rheumatoid nodules, if present, aid in the diagnosis.

- For oligoarticular disease, osteoarthritis can pose a diagnostic challenge. However, age group, bone mineral density, non-inflammatory signs and classic radiograph findings of the large joints like knees and hip will help to make the correct diagnosis.

- Joint inflammation may also be seen in a septic joint but palpating the joint reveals a hot, tender and tense joint and joint fluid aspiration followed by culture will reveal the causative organism.
- Dactylitis with sausage-shaped fingers and uncontrolled disease resulting in joint destruction may also be seen in systemic lupus erythematosus (SLE). Cutaneous findings of SLE rash on photoexposed areas, features of vasculitis and a positive ANA, point to SLE with joint involvement.

Diagnostic Criteria

The first diagnostic criteria was proposed by Moll and Wright in 1973. It required the patient to have psoriasis, a negative rheumatid factor and the presence of inflammatory arthritis in any of 5 clinical patterns. Although simple and highly specific, the criteria lacks sensitivity in diagnosing PsA. In 2006, the Classification of Psoriatic Arthritis (CASPAR) criteria were published which have high sensitivity and specificity.[19] The criteria require the presence of inflammatory articular disease (joint, spine, or entheseal) with ≥3 points from the following categories:

- Evidence of current psoriasis (2 points)
- A personal past history or family history of psoriasis (1 point)
- Psoriatic nail dystrophy (1 point)
- Dactylitis (1 point)
- Negative RA test (1 point)
- Radiograph showing juxta-articular new bone formation (1 point)

The CASPAR criterion is widely used because it helps to identify patients with early disease irrespective of their ethnicity.

Once a diagnosis is made and treatment initiated, the change in disease process must be evaluated to monitor treatment efficacy and predict disease outcome. Various criteria have been formulated and include:

- American College of Rheumatology 20% improvement (ARC20)
- Psoriatic Arthritis Response Criteria (PsARC)
- Disease Activity Score in 28 joints (DAS28)
- European League Against Rheumatism (EULAR) response criteria
- Group for Research and Assessment of Psoriasis and Psoriatic Arthritis (GRAPPA)

Management

Traditionally considered as a sero-negative arthropathy, the treatment protocols were based on similar lines as rheumatid arthritis. Non-steroidal anti-inflammatory drugs (NSAIDs) were considered first line followed by steroids and synthetic disease modifying anti-rheumatic drugs (DMRDs). However, with better understanding of the disease process and the introduction of biologics, there has been a dramatic change in the management and thus the disease outcome in PsA.[20, 21] The change has been from providing relief from joint pains by reducing joint destruction and preventing disability.

NSAIDs

Nimesulide 200 or 400 mg/day has been effectively used to reduce musculoskeletal symptoms in early and mild disease. But its disadvantages appear to be greater, presenting as adverse drug reactions in the form of gastrointestinal and renal toxicity. Cardiovascular disturbances have also been reported. Also, these drugs have no effect on psoriatic plaques.

Corticosteroids

Systemic corticosteroids are effective but are associated with significant flare-up of disease upon stopping and have been reported to precipitate pustular psoriasis. Mahajan and colleagues have proposed the use of low-dose corticosteroids combined with DMARDs as a good therapeutic option to reduce inflammation and joint destruction.[22] Intra-lesional/articular steroids have been used with variable success when isolated joints are involved or when combined with systemic therapy as an adjuvant.

DMARDs

- Methotrexate (MTX):
  - Till recently, MTX was considered the first line treatment for the management of PsA. At doses of 15 mg/week and higher, it improves the PASI score and provides relief in peripheral joint disease. However, with more studies and data available, it has not shown to be of any benefit in treating axial diseases. It is not effective in reducing synovitis and enthesitis in patients, thereby questioning its long-term use and use as a first line modality in treating PsA.

- Cyclosporine
  - Inhibiting T-cell activation, it is a rapid and effective drug for skin lesions but its efficacy in PsA is not proven. It has been used in the dose of 3–5 mg/kg/day in divided doses. It has also been combined with MTX and TNF-α inhibitors for improved efficacy. However, the side effect profile prevents its long-term use.

- Leflunomide
  - This pyrimidine synthetase inhibitor has shown very promising results in improving joint disease and clearing skin lesions. In patients refractory to MTX therapy, leflunomide has shown to improve symptoms. It has been started with a loading dose of 100 mg/day for 3 days followed by 20 mg/day. However, it is a category X drug with a washout period of up to 2 years. Hence should be used with caution in women of child-bearing potential.

- Sulfasalazine
  - This drug has shown to improve joint function in PsA but its ability to stop disease progression is not validated. When combined with MTX, it improves overall efficacy but altered liver enzymes and hence can be a limiting factor. It is started at a 1.5 g/day in divided doses and gradually increased to 4 g/day.

Biologics

Biologics have revolutionized the treatment of PsA as they have been successful in curtailing the inflammation, preventing the extension of joint damage, and giving immense relief in pain management. Biologics are the only agents which give relief for dactylitis, enthesitis and spondyloarthritis.

Biologics target various components in the inflammatory pathway of psoriasis, viz. TNF, IL-23, IL-17, IL-6, CTLA-4, PDE4 and others.

Tumor Necrosis Factor (TNF) inhibitors include infliximab, etanercept, adalimumab, golimumab and certolizumabpegol. Since these agents aim at blocking TNF at various events in the inflammatory pathway, the efficacy is similar, except for the latest entrant-certolizumabpegol. It has a significantly higher ARC20 response at 12 weeks as compared to others. A comparative study of etanercept, infliximab and adalimumab in 100 patients of PsA showed favorable outcome for all 3 drugs.[23]

Interleukin-12/23 Inhibitor: Ustekinumab[24]

This human monoclonal antibody binds to the common subunit p40 of IL-12 and IL-23. It is safe and well tolerated and has the advantage of inhibiting progression of joint damage as seen on pre- and post-treatment radiographs. It is administered as 45 mg or 90 mg subcutaneous injections at weeks 0, 4 and every 12 weeks thereafter.

Phosphodiesterase Inhibitor (PDE4): Apremilast[25]

PDE4 is responsible for degradation of cyclic adenosine monophosphate (cAMP). Its inhibition results in intracellular accumulation of cAMP which downregulates production of pro-inflammatory cytokines and upregulates release of anti-inflammatory cytokines like IL-10. It has to be taken orally with doses of 20–40 mg twice daily. It has shown good efficacy with a very high safety profile not requiring any routine lab monitoring.

Interleukin-17 inhibitors include secukinumab, ixekuzumab and brodalumab. Although their role in reducing skin and nail psoriasis has been shown, their effectiveness in PsA needs further evaluation.

JAK Inhibitors: Tofacitinib

It inhibits JAK3 and JAK1, thereby blocking release of pro-inflammatory cytokines like IL-2, IL-4, IL-15 and IL-21. Their use in PsA is under trials.

The cost of biological therapy has been the point of concern for most due to prohibitive costs and unknown duration of therapy. However, detailed and systematic economic analysis of biological therapy (TNFi) for early, active PsA has shown to be cost-effective compared to conventional line of treatment.[26] Etanercept has been shown to be most cost-effective as compared to other biologicals.

Treatment in Pregnancy and Lactation

Case reports of PsA associated with pregnancy are rare. The therapeutic options are significantly restricted and safety profile of many new drugs has not been evaluated. The ones which have shown to be safe or have a low risk profile include sulfasalazine and cyclosporine, in reduced dosage. Oral corticosteroids can be used. Azathioprine has been reported to cause premature births but not congenital defects.

The use of biologics is not advocated due to limited or no data available. Congenital malformations have been reported with the use of etanercept, infliximab and adalimumab during pregnancy.[27]

CONCLUSION

Psoriatic arthritis is increasingly being recognized as an independent and distinct arthropathy with inflammation, joint destruction and significant impairment in quality of life. As dermatologist, we can identify probable cases with early disease so that early and effective therapy can be initiated to improve clinical outcome in the long run.

REFERENCES

1. Kumar R, Sharma A, Dogra S. Prevalence and clinical patterns of psoriatic arthritis in Indian patients with psoriasis. Indian J Dermatol Venereol Leprol 2014;80:15–23.

2. Gladman DD. Psoriatic arthritis from Wright's era until today. J Rheumatol 2009;83:4–8.

3. Budu-Aggrey A, Bowes J, Barton A. Identifying a novel locus for psoriatic arthritis. Rheumatology (Oxford). 2015 Aug 8,pii: kev273.

4. Fitzgerald O, Haroon M, Giles JT, Winchester R. Concepts of pathogenesis in psoriatic arthritis: genotype determines clinical phenotype. Arthritis Res Ther 2015 May 7;17:115.

5. Kumar R, Sharma A, Dogra S. Prevalence and clinical patterns of psoriatic arthritis in Indian patients with psoriasis. Indian J Dermatol Venereol Leprol 2014;80:15–23.

6. Peluso R, Iervolino S, Vitiello M, Bruner V, Lupoli G, Di Minno MN. Extra-articular manifestations in psoriatic arthritis patients. ClinRheumatol 2015 Apr;34(4):745–53.

7. Restrepo JP, Medina LF, Molina Mdel P. Peripheral corneal melting syndrome in psoriatic arthritis treated with adalimumab. Rev Bras Reumatol 2015 Jul-Aug;55(4):387–9.

8. Dogra A, Arora AK. Nail psoriasis: the journey so far. Indian J Dermatol. 2014 Jul;59(4):319–33.

9. Prasad PV, Bikku B, Kaviarasan PK, Senthilnathan A. A clinical study of psoriatic arthropathy. Indian J Dermatol Venereol Leprol. 2007 May-Jun;73(3):166–70.

10. Aydin SZ, Castillo-Gallego C, Ash ZR, Marzo-Ortega H, Emery P, Wakefield RJ, et al. Ultrasonographic assessment of nail in psoriatic disease shows a link between onychopathy and distal interphalangeal

joint extensor tendon enthesopathy. Dermatology 2012;225(3): 231–5.

11. McGonagle D. Enthesitis: an autoinflammatory lesion linking nail and joint involvement in psoriatic disease. J Eur Acad Dermatol Venereol. 2009 Sep;23(Suppl 1):9–13.

12. Ahn CS, Dothard EH, Garner ML, Feldman SR, Huang WW. To test or not to test? An updated evidence-based assessment of the value of screening and monitoring tests when using systemic biologic agents to treat psoriasis and psoriatic arthritis. J Am Acad Dermatol 2015 Sep; 73(3):420–428.e1.

13. Chandran V, Scher JU. Biomarkers in psoriatic arthritis: recent progress. Curr Rheumatol Rep 2014 Nov;16(11):453.

14. De Simone C, Guerriero C, Giampetruzzi AR, Costantini M, Di Gregorio F, Amerio P. Achilles tendinitis in psoriasis: clinical and sonographic findings. J Am AcadDermatol 2003 Aug;49(2):217–22.

15. Lin Z1, Wang Y, Mei Y, Zhao Y, Zhang Z. High-frequency ultrasound in the evaluation of psoriatic arthritis: A clinical study. Am J Med Sci 2015 Jul;350(1):42–6.

16. Gutierrez M, Filippucci E, De Angelis R, Salaffi F, Filosa G, Ruta S, et al. Subclinical entheseal involvement in patients with psoriasis: an ultrasound study. Semin Arthritis Rheum 2011 Apr;40(5):407–12.

17. Narváez J1, Narváez JA, de Albert M, Gómez-Vaquero C, Nolla JM. Can magnetic resonance imaging of the hand and wrist differentiate between rheumatoid arthritis and psoriatic arthritis in the early stages of the disease? Semin Arthritis Rheum 2012 Dec;42(3):234–45.

18. Coates LC, Hodgson R, Conaghan PG, Freeston JE. MRI and ultra-sonography for diagnosis and monitoring of psoriatic arthritis. Best Pract Res Clin Rheumatol 2012 Dec;26(6):805–22.

19. Zlatkovic-Svenda M, Kerimovic-Morina D, Stojanovic RM. Psoriatic arthritis classification criteria: Moll and Wright, ESSG and CASPAR — a comparative study. ActaReumatol Port 2013 Jul–Sep;38(3):172–8.

20. Kang EJ, Kavanaugh A. Psoriatic arthritis: latest treatments and their place in therapy. TherAdv Chronic Dis 2015 Jul;6(4):194–203.

21. Sritheran D, Leung YY. Making the next steps in psoriatic arthritis management: current status and future directions. Ther Adv Musculo-skelet Dis 2015 Oct;7(5):173–86.

22. Mahajan VK, Sharma AL, Chauhan PS, Mehta KS, Sharma NL. Early treatment with addition of low dose prednisolone to methotrexate improves therapeutic outcome in severe psoriatic arthritis. Indian J Dermatol 2013 May;58(3):240.

23. Atteno M, Peluso R, Costa L, Padula S, Iervolino S, Caso F, et al. Comparison of effectiveness and safety of infliximab, etanercept, and adalimumab in psoriatic arthritis patients who experienced an inadequate response to previous disease-modifying antirheumatic drugs. ClinRheumatol 2010 Apr;29(4):399–403.

24. Kavanaugh A, Ritchlin C, Rahman P, Puig L, Gottlieb AB, Li S, et al. Ustekinumab, an anti-IL-12/23 p40 monoclonal antibody, inhibits radiographic progression in patients with active psoriatic arthritis: Results of an integrated analysis of radiographic data from the phase 3, multicentre, randomised, double-blind, placebo-controlled PSUMMIT-1 and PSUMMIT-2 trials. Ann Rheum Dis 2014 Jun;73(6): 1000–6.

25. Abdulrahim H1, Thistleton S, Adebajo AO, Shaw T, Edwards C, Wells A. Apremilast: a PDE4 inhibitor for the treatment of psoriatic arthritis. Expert OpinPharmacother 2015 May;16(7):1099–108.

26. Cawson MR, Mitchell SA, Knight C, Wildey H, Spurden D, Bird A, et al. Systematic review, network meta-analysis and economic evaluation of biological therapy for the management of active psoriatic arthritis. BMC Musculoskelet Disord 2014 Jan 20;15:26.

27. Kurizky PS, Ferreira Cde C, Nogueira LS, da Mota LM. Treatment of psoriasis and psoriatic arthritis during pregnancy and breastfeeding. An Bras Dermatol 2015 May-Jun;90(3):367–75.

11

Topical Therapies in Psoriasis

Manjyot M Gautam

INTRODUCTION

In India, prevalence of psoriasis varies from 0.44 to 2.8%. Majority of these patients have mild to moderate disease and can be treated with topical agents which provide potential therapeutic efficacy and limit the effects of the treatment to the target tissue.

INDICATIONS

Topical therapy is the treatment of choice in patients with psoriasis affecting less than 10% body surface area (BSA).

It can also be used for the treatment of psoriasis in sensitive areas like the face, flexures and genitals.

Topical agents are also used as adjuvant for:

- Psoriasis affecting >10% BSA who are being concurrently treated with either phototherapy or systemic medications
- Refractory palmoplantar psoriasis
- Resistant scalp psoriasis
- Patients with significant psychosocial impairment

FACTORS WHICH DETERMINE TREATMENT

Patient Factors

Treatment must be individualized according to the patient's age, sex, occupation, understanding, affordability and the available resources.

Disease Factors

Treatment will also depend on the site of the lesions, their extent and severity.

Vehicle

There are a vast array of vehicles including creams, gels, solutions, foams, sprays, shampoos and lotions. The choice of the vehicle depends upon the sites involved. Gels, solutions or foams are preferred for scalp psoriasis. Elsewhere, patients may prefer a less greasy preparation like a cream during the daytime and use an ointment which is more effective but less cosmetically appealing at night.

Occlusion

Occlusion therapy enhances the penetration of topical agents such as corticosteroids. The occlusive dressings trap heat and moisture, hydrating and macerating the skin and forcing the medication through the plaques.

Combination Therapy

Combination therapy is indicated when monotherapy with topical agents is inadequate or to prevent or reduce the side effects of topical agents. For example, the combination of superpotent steroids and calcipotriene. However, when using multiple topical agents, it is important to be aware of possible compatibility issues, for example, salicylic acid inactivates calcipotriene. On the other hand, anthralin requires salicylic acid for its chemical stability. When it is desirable to use multiple topical agents, patients may be instructed to apply the various medications at separate times throughout the day.

EMOLLIENTS AND MOISTURIZERS

Emollients and moisturizers form the backbone of therapy for psoriasis. They should be combined with other topical therapies during the active stage of the disease. Once the patient goes into remission, emollients alone can be used for maintenance.

Mechanism of Action

Emollients and moisturizers help in normalizing hyper-proliferation, differentiation, and apoptosis and inflammation, thus improve the barrier function and provide and retain hydration of the stratum corneum. This makes the epidermis more resistant to external stress and reduces the induction of Koebner's phenomenon.

Besides helping the skin to retain water, emollients:

- Moisturise dry skin
- Ease itching
- Reduce scaling
- Soften cracks
- Allow other topical treatments to enter the skin

Vehicles and Preparations

Emollients are available as creams, ointments, lotion, bath oils and soap substitutes. Creams and ointments are preferable to lotions as they tend to be thicker, more occlusive and therefore more effective. Ointments are more suited for extra dry, thickened or brittle skin and can be used at night. Lighter, less greasy creams or lotions are ideal for daytime use.

The commonly used emollients are petroleum jelly, liquid paraffin and mineral oils.

Adverse Effects

Emollients can cause a few side effects, such as irritant dermatitis, allergic contact dermatitis, fragrance allergy or allergy to other constituents, stinging, cosmetic acne and pigmentary disorders.

TOPICAL CORTICOSTEROIDS

Topical corticosteroids (TCS) are universally used in the management of all grades of psoriasis. They are used as monotherapy when the disease is mild and as adjuvants to systemic therapy in patients with moderate to severe psoriasis.

Mechanism of Action

Corticosteroids are vasoconstrictive, anti-proliferative, anti-inflammatory and immunosuppressive. These effects are mediated through their binding to intracellular corticosteroid receptor and regulation of gene transcription of numerous genes, particularly those that code for pro-inflammatory cytokines.

Potency of TCS

They are available in varying strengths, ranging from the lowest potency class 7 steroids to the superpotent class 1 steroids.

Potent and superpotent TCS may be used for stubborn, thick, chronic plaques (Table 11.1).

Table 11.1: Selecting potency of TCS and vehicle according to the site involved

Site	Potency of TCS	Vehicle
Face	Low and medium potency	Creams
Intertriginous areas	Low and medium potency	Creams
Trunk and extremities	Moderate to potent	Ointment, spray, foam
Palms and soles	Potent to superpotent	Ointment
Scalp	Moderate to high	Solution, lotion, foam, gel, shampoo

Adverse Effects

Long-term use of TCS can lead to tachyphylaxis—the loss of effectiveness or the development of resistance to TCS over approximately 2–4 months. However, many psoriasis experts have challenged this phenomenon and claim that tachyphylaxis merely represents a decline in patient adherence to therapy and not a decline in efficacy.

Systemic adverse events occur when TCS are used for prolonged periods of time or at doses higher than commonly prescribed (Table 11.2).

Gradual withdrawal of TCS is recommended to avoid this rebound phenomenon.

TCS, particularly when used in high doses, can lead to a pustular flare of psoriasis when discontinued.

Table 11.2: Side effects of TCS involved

Cutaneous side-effects	Systemic side-effects
Skin atrophy	Suppression of HPA axis
Striae	Adrenal suppression
Pigmentary changes	Hyperglycemia
Hypertrichosis	Avascular necrosis of femoral head
Telangiectasias	Cushing's syndrome
Allergic contact dermatitis	
Easy bruising, purpura	
Increased susceptibility to infections	
Rebound phenomenon	
Perioral dermatitis	

TCS Use in Pregnancy and in Pediatric Population

- TCS are labeled as category C in pregnancy. Their safety in breast feeding is unknown.

Infants and young children are at greater risk for side-effects. Both growth retardation and suppression of the HPA axis have been documented in children more frequently. Also class 1 TCS should not be used in children less than 12 years of age.

New Vehicle Formulations for TCS

Are available in shampoos, sprays and in foam preparations.

Recommendation of TCS

- Once clinical improvement occurs, the frequency of application should be reduced.
- For maintenance, TCS can be used intermittently (weekends).
- If the lesions are very thick when continuous application of class 1 TCS can be extended beyond 3 weeks with a maximum weekly dose of 30 g.

VITAMIN D ANALOGS

Vitamin D analogs provide a useful adjunct in the treatment of chronic plaque psoriasis.

Mechanism of Action

Vitamin D analogs bind to the intracellular vitamin D receptor which then binds to and regulates genes involved in epidermal proliferation, inflammation and keratinization.

There are three vitamin D analog preparations available to treat psoriasis: calcipotriene (calcipotriol in Europe), calcitriol and tacalcitol.

Efficacy

Vitamin D analogs are safe and effective in the treatment of chronic plaque psoriasis. They have similar efficacy to class 2 and 3 TCS but relatively fewer side effects. In comparison to superpotent TCS, their onset of action is delayed but results in longer disease free interval.

As monotherapy, vitamin D analogs are recommended in psoriasis affecting a BSA ≤10%.

Calcipotriene is available as 0.005% (5 micrograms/gram) cream, ointment and scalp lotion.

Calcitriol is available as an ointment only (3 micrograms/gram). Tacalcitol is available as 4 micrograms/gram ointment and lotion.

Calcipotriene and calcitriol need to be applied twice daily, whereas tacalcitol has an added advantage of once daily application.

Calcitriol and tacalcitol, being less irritating, are preferred over calcipotriene, for lesions on the face and intertriginous areas. The maximum recommended dose of calcipotriene is 100 g/wk, calcitriol is 200 g/wk and tacalcitol is 70 g/wk. The safety of calcipotriene and calcitriol has been established for a period of 52 weeks and 78 weeks respectively.

Vitamin D analogs can also be used in combination with potent TCS in the form of sequential therapy.

Adverse Effects

The most common adverse effect is skin irritation on or around the psoriasis plaques especially face and intertriginous area. Calcitriol and tacalcitol have a better tolerability on sensitive areas as compared to calcipotriene.

Systemic side effects like hypercalcemia, hypercalciuria and parathyroid hormone suppression are very rare.

Calcitriol may have greater effects on serum calcium in comparison to other analogs.

Vitamin D analogs are contraindicated in patients already suffering from hypercalcemia. Patients with renal impairment need to be observed carefully.

Calcipotriene is a relatively unstable molecule that is inactivated by an acid pH, therefore should not be used in combination with salicylic acid.

When combined with phototherapy, calcipotriene should be applied following phototherapy.

Topical Vitamin D Analog use in Pregnancy and Pediatric Population

Vitamin D analogs are rated category C in pregnancy. Use of calcipotriene for the treatment of psoriasis in children is effective and the dose should not exceed 50 g/wk in children between 6 and 12 years of age and 75 g/wk in children more than 12 years old.

Topical Vitamin D Analog use in Nursing Mothers

It is not known whether calcipotriene is excreted in human milk. So caution should be exercised in a nursing woman.

TOPICAL IMMUNOMODULATORS

Topical Calcineurin Inhibitors (TCI)

There are no FDA approved indications for psoriasis. Tacrolimus (0.03% and 0.1%) and pimecrolimus cream (1%) can be used for the treatment of facial and intertriginous psoriasis.

Mechanism of Action

Calcineurin inhibitors inhibit the action of calcineurin phosphatase and block the production of inflammatory substances.

Both tacrolimus and pimecrolimus are effective in treating psoriasis, where the skin is thin, i.e. on the face, genitalia and intertriginous areas.

Penetration can also be improved by combining these agents with salicylic acid.

Efficacy

In a randomized, controlled trial, topical tacrolimus 0.3% gel was found to be equivalent to 0.005% calcipotriol ointment for treatment of mild-to-moderate plaque psoriasis. However, calcipotriol treated lesions had a faster rate of improvement.

They are applied twice a day to the affected areas. However, the duration of course is not specified.

Adverse Effects

The most common adverse events with tacrolimus and pimecrolimus are stinging and/or pruritus seen within the first few days of treatment. These symptoms tend to diminish with ongoing use.

Topical immunomodulators should not be used as long-term treatment, over large surface areas, or in children under the age of two years.

Use of Calcineurin Inhibitors in Pregnancy and Pediatric Population

Topical tacrolimus and pimecrolimus are pregnancy category C. Both these medicines are found in human milk, thus not recommended for nursing mothers.

TAZAROTENE

Tazarotene, a vitamin A derivative, is available as a gel or cream at concentration of 0.1% or 0.05%.

It is indicated for stable plaque psoriasis but is usually prescribed in combination with other therapies for psoriasis like TCS and calcipotriene and is effective as maintenance therapy for psoriasis.

It is recommended that treatment commences with 0.05% formulation to avoid irritation and the concentration increased if necessary.

Tazarotene is applied once a day in the evening.

Mechanism of Action

Tazarotene selectively binds to β and γ retinoic acid on the cell membrane of keratinocytes and is then transported to the nucleus, altering transcription of genes in keratinocytes. This results in reduced epidermal hyperproliferation, normalizing keratinocyte differentiation and decreasing inflammation.

Adverse Effects

The most common side effect of tazarotene is localized irritation. The use of cream, low concentration, alternate day application and short contact (30–60 mins) application may help alleviate such symptoms.

Concomitant use of topical corticosteroids may also minimize symptoms.

The FDA has issued a caution regarding the use of tazarotene and exposure to sunlight and patients are advised to use sunscreens when using tazarotene. In cases when the agent is used in combination with phototherapy, the dosimetry might need to be lowered to prevent skin burning.

Use of Tazarotene in Pregnancy and in Pediatric Patients

Tazarotene is pregnancy category X.

Children tolerate topical retinoids very well. Topical retinoids are therefore considered safe and efficacious in the pediatric populations.

ANTHRALIN (DITHRANOL)

Anthralin is the synthetic version of chrysarobin, a product derived from the araroba tree in South America.

Mechanism of Action

The exact mechanism of action is unclear. Anthralin reduces keratinocyte proliferation, prevents T cell activation and restores cell differentiation, probably through mitochondrial dysfunction.

Modes of Application of Anthralin

Anthralin can be applied either as overnight application of anthralin to involved areas followed by UVB therapy (Ingram regimen), or as short contact anthralin therapy (SCAT) in which high concentrations of anthralin 1% or greater is applied for minutes to an hour prior to removal.

Adverse Effects

The most common side effect of anthralin is skin irritation which is dose related. It should be applied with caution to face and intertriginous areas.

It also stains lesional and adjoining skin, hair, nails, clothing and other objects with which patients come into contact. Triethanolamine applied after the removal of anthralin, prevents staining and irritation by neutralizing any anthralin residue remaining on the skin.

No systemic toxicity has been reported even following long term application of anthralin.

Anthralin is pregnancy category C.

Children: Use with caution.

Salicylic acid is frequently added to improve the stability of anthralin and to increase its penetration and efficacy.

Preparations

Dithranol is available as:

1. Derobin ointment containing dithranol 1.15%, coal tar solution 5.3 %, salicylic acid 1.15%, petrolatum base.
2. Micanol is a 1% anthralin formulation in a temperature sensitive vehicle (microcapsules). It is particularly useful for scalp psoriasis.
3. Liposomal Dithranol formulation (lipogel) is as efficacious as the conventional preparation but is much less irritating and much less staining than the latter.

COAL TAR

It is the liquid by-product of coal distillation. It is a mixture of hydrocarbons with different components such as benzols, naphthalene and anthralenes. Coal tar is frequently used as a part of an inpatient or daily dressing regimen. Its use in conjunction with UVB, the Goeckerman regimen, is well recognised.

Mechanism of Action

The mode of action of coal tar is not precisely known, although it clearly has anti-proliferative actions. This is probably through suppression of DNA synthesis, thereby reducing the hyper-proliferative state of keratinocytes.

Side Effects

Adverse effects of coal tar include odor, staining, irritant contact dermatitis, erythema, stinging, folliculitis and formation of keratoacanthomas.

Occupational coal tar exposure is a recognised carcinogen.

Treatment with PUVA and coal tar is not recommended and has been estimated to produce a 2–4 fold increase in risk of skin cancer.

Coal tar may be used during pregnancy.

Coal tar should be used with caution in the pediatric population.

Newer Formulations of Coal Tar

Modifications have been made to tar preparations to reduce its side effects and to increase its acceptability. These new formulations are cosmetically elegant.

1. *Exorex*: It contains coal tar 1%. It has the advantage of rapid penetration and absence of staining and smell.
2. *Scytera*: It is an emollient foam containing 10% coal tar topical solution (liquor carbonis detergens) equivalent to 2 % coal tar. It offers advantages of easy spreadability and uses a patented odor neutralizing system to minimize the coal tar odor.
3. *Liquor carbonis distillate (LCD) 15% solution*: LCD is a solution equivalent to 2.3% coal tar. It uses an evaporative and transparent vehicle for rapid absorption, fragrance and dab-on applicator.

SALICYLIC ACID

Salicylic acid is a topical keratolytic agent.

Mode of Action

Salicylic acid leads to desquamation of corneocyctes through two pathways. It reduces intercellular cohesiveness of the horny cells by dissolving the intercellular cement material. It also reduces the pH of the stratum corneum, thereby increasing hydration and softening.

Efficacy

Salicylic acid is often combined with other topical agents, including topical corticosteroids and immunomodulators in the therapy of psoriasis. Salicylic acid greatly increases the penetration rate of topical corticosteroids because of its keratolytic effects.

Steroid—salicylic acid combination can be used as first line of treatment on thick, scaly plaques.

Salicylic acid can be applied to areas with thick stratum corneum including palms, soles, and scalp. It can also be used on the trunk. Its use should be avoided on genitals, the mucous membrane and the eyes.

The addition of salicylic acid to dithranol formulations improves the clinical efficacy of dithranol because of the antioxidant properties of salicylic acid.

It can be applied as a paste or in creams, ointments, lotions in concentration of 2–6%.

Adverse Effects

The major problem in the topical treatment of psoriasis with salicylic acid is the risk of salicylism. Therefore, salicylic acid should not be applied to more than 20% of the body surface area.

Some topical treatments of psoriasis, such as calcipotriol, are inactivated by salicylic acid.

It should be noted that salicylic acid should be applied after phototherapy, as it blocks ultraviolet light.

Pregnancy and Children

Salicylic acid can be safely used for localized psoriasis in pregnancy; however, because of a greater risk of systemic absorption and toxicity, salicylic acid should be avoided in the treatment of children less than 6 years of age.

COMBINATION THERAPY

The commonly used topical medications for psoriasis achieve efficacy through different mechanisms which provides a potential rationale for combination therapy. Combination topical therapies are frequently used in clinical practice for patients with mild to moderate psoriasis. Data from a number of clinical trials suggest that combination therapies may have greater efficacy, tolerability, and, perhaps, fewer combined adverse effects compared with monotherapies.

Vitamin D Analogues and Corticosteroid

Vitamin D analogue—with class 1 or 2 corticosteroid combination is more effective in inducing disease clearance.

Sequential Therapy

Induction phase: A class 1 corticosteroid in the morning and calcipotriene at night. As an alternative, combination of calcipotriene with betamethasone dipropionate in a single ointment base can also be applied twice daily during this stage. This phase usually lasts 2–4 weeks.

Transition phase: During this period, TCS use is restricted to weekends only (2 days) while calcipotriene is applied on weekdays (5 days). This is also called pulse therapy or weekday-weekend therapy, length of this phase may vary from 1 to 6 months.

Maintenance phase: TCS is discontinued altogether; calcipotriene is used for long-term maintenance.

Vitamin D Analogues and UV-B

Combination of vitamin D analogue with UV-B is not more effective than UV-B monotherapy. However, the combination is more efficacious than vitamin D analogue monotherapy.

Vitamin D Analogues and Tazarotene

Combination of vitamin D analogues with tazarotene may be an effective alternative to steroid based regimens.

Corticosteroid and Salicylic Acid

The combination of topical corticosteroids and salicylic acid may be valuable as salicylic acid greatly increases the penetration rate of topical corticosteroids because of its keratolytic effect.

However, a recent meta-analysis demonstrated that combination of topical steroid and salicylic acid was not more effective than topical corticosteroid monotherapy.

Tacrolimus and Salicylic Acid

The combination of tacrolimus with salicylic acid is more efficacious than tacrolimus monotherapy as salicylic acid increases the penetration of tacrolimus.

RECOMMENDED READING

1. Alora-Palli MB, Perkins AC, Van Cott A, Kimball AB. Efficacy and tolerability of a cosmetically acceptable coal tar solution in the treatment of moderate plaque psoriasis: A controlled comparison with calcipotriol cream. J Clin Dermatol 2010;11(4):275–83.

2. Bailey EE, Ference EH, Alikhan A, Meghan T. Hession MT, Armstrong AW. Combination of topical therapies: Combination Treatments for Psoriasis: A Systematic Review and Meta-analysis.Arch Dermatol. 2012;148(4):511–22.

3. Brune A, Miller DW, Lin P, Cotrim-Russi D, Paller AS. Tacrolimus ointment is effective for psoriasis on face and intertriginous areas in pediatric patients. Pediatr Dermatol 2007;24(1)76–80.

4. Bruner CR, Feldman SR, Ventapragada M, Fleischer AB Jr. A systematic review of adverse effects associated with topical treatments for psoriasis. Dermatol Online J 2003;9:2.

5. Chi C-C, Wang S-H, Kirtschig G, Wojnarowska F. Systematic review of the safety of topical corticosteroids in pregnancy. J Am Acad Dermatol 2010;62:694–705.

6. Devaux S, Castela A, Archier E, Gallini A, Joly P, Misery L, Aractingi S, Aubin F, Bachelez H, Cribier B, Jullien D, Le Maître M, Richard MA, Ortonne JP, Paul C. Topical vitamin D analogues alone or in association with topical steroids for psoriasis: A systematic review. JEADV 2012;26:52–60.

7. Fluhr JW, Cavallotti C, Berardesca E. Emollients, moisturizers and keratolytic agents in psoriasis. Clin Dermatol 2008;26(4):380–6.

8. Frankel AJ, Zeichner JA, Del Rosso JQ. Coal tar 2% foam in combination with a superpotent corticosteroid for chronic plaque psoriasis. J Clin Aesthet Dermatol 2010;3(10):42–5.

9. Guenther L, Van de Kerkhof PC, Snellman E, et al. Efficacy and safety of a new combination of calcipotriol and betamethasone dipropionate (once or twice daily) compared to calcipotriol (twice daily) in the treatment of psoriasis vulgaris: A randomized, double blind, vehicle controlled clinical trial. Br J Dermatol 2002;147:316–23.

10. Hengge UR, Ruzicka T, Schwartz RA, Cork MJ. Adverse effects of topical glucocorticoids. J Am Acad Dermatol 2006;54:1–15.

11. Jemec GB, Ganslandt C, Ortonne JP, Poulin Y, Burden AD, de Unamono P, et al. A new scalp formulation of calcipotriol plus betamethasone compared with its active ingredients and the vehicle in the treatment of scalp psoriasis: A randomized, double- blind controlled trial. J Am Acad Dermatol 2008;59:455–63.

12. Kane D, Barnes L, Fitzgerald O. Topical corticosteroid therapy: Systemic side effects. British J Dermatol 2003;149:417.

13. Kircik L. Efficacy and safety of topical calcitriol 3 micrograms/gram ointment, a new topical therapy for chronic plaque psoriasis. J Drugs Dermatol 2009;8(8 Suppl):S9–S16.

14. Koo JY. New developments in topical sequential therapy for psoriasis. Skin Therapy Lett 2005 Nov;10(9):1–4.

15. Koo JY. Using topical multimodal strategies for patients with psoriasis. Cutis 2007;79(1)(Suppl 2):11–17.

16. Lam J, Polifka JE, Dohil MA. Safety of dermatologic drugs used in pregnancy patients with psoriasis and other inflammatory skin diseases. J Am Acad Dermatol 2008;59:295–315.

17. Lebwohl M, Ali S. Treatment of Psoriasis. Part 1. Topical treatment and phototherapy. J Am Acad Dermatol 2001;45:487–98.

18. Marsland AM, Griffiths CE. The macrolide immunosuppressants in dermatology. Mechanism of action. Eur J Dermatol 2002;12:618–22.

19. Mehta BH, Amladi SK. Evaluation of topical 0.1% tazarotene cream in the treatment of palmoplantar psoriasis: an observer blinded randomized controlled trial 2011;56:40–3.

20. Menter A, Korman NJ, Elmets CA, et al. Guidelines of care for the management of psoriasis or psoriatic arthritis. Section 3. Guidelines of care for the management of psoriasis with topical therapies. J Am Acad Dermatol 2009;60:643–59.

21. Paul C, Gallini A, Archier E, Castela E, Devaux S, et al. Evidence-based recommendations on topical treatment and phototherapy of psoriasis: systematic review and expert opinion of a panel of Dermatologists. JEADV 2012;26(Suppl 3):1–10.

22. Poulin Y, Papp K, Bissonnette R, et al. Clobetasol propionate shampoo 0.05% is efficacious and safe for long-term control of moderate scalp psoriasis. J Dermatolog Treat 2010;21(3):185–92.

23. Van de Kerkhof PC, Barker J, Griffiths CE et al. Psoriasis consensus on topical therapies. J Eur Acad Dermatol Venereol 2008;22:859–70.

24. Veraldi S, Caputo R, Pacifico A, et al. Short contact therapy with tazarotene in psoriasis vulgaris. Dermatology 2006;212:235–7.

12

Systemic Therapies in Psoriasis

Parag Sharma

Broad spectrums of antipsoriatic treatment are available which are mostly immunomodulatory. When choosing a treatment we should consider the extent and severity of the disease, patients own perception of the disease and safety of the treatment.[1]

The antipsoriatic drugs can be classified by their mechanism of action as follows:

i. *Antimitotics*: Methotrexate, hydroxyurea, thioguanine, mycophenolate mofetil, fumaric acid esters.

ii. *Immunosuppressives*: Cyclosporine, biologicals
   - *Anti IL-2*: Cyclosporine, alefacept, efazulimab.
   - Anti-TNF-α: Etanercept, infliximab, adalimumab.

iii. *Anti-proliferative and anti-inflammatory*: Retinoids, calcitriol.

As the antipsoriatic drugs are immunomodulatory, they share many features. So in this chapter the common features of all the drugs will be discussed and their specific features will be highlighted.

MECHANISM OF ACTION

The antimitotics inhibits nucleotides, thereby reducing DNA synthesis. Methotrexate suppresses thymine and purine nucleotides by inhibiting dihydrofolate reductase enzyme (inhibits cell division in S phase). Mycophenolate mofetil blocks synthesis of guanine. Thioguanine interferes with purine biosynthesis. Hydroxyurea inhibits the M_2 subunit of Ribonucleotide reductase (inhibits cell division in G_2 phase). Fumaric acid esters inhibit keratinocyte proliferation.[1]

The antimitotics also have anti-inflammatory actions. Methotrexate decreases inflammation by increasing adenosine (anti-inflammatory mediator) and decreasing S-adenyl methionine (pro-inflammatory mediator).[2] Hydroxyurea causes hypomethylation of genes inducing differentiation and normalization of psoriatic skin.[3] Mycophenolate mofetil decreases immunoglobulin levels and suppresses antibody formation by B lymphocytes. Fumaric acid esters changes Th1 dominated T-cell response to Th2 pattern.[1]

Cyclosporine, alefacept and efazulimab prevent T-cell activation. Cyclosporine, a calcineurin inhibitor, prevents T-lymphocyte activation from being translated into the release of IL-2. This results in decrease in the number of CD4$^+$ and CD8$^+$ T-cells in epidermis.[4] Alefacept binds to CD2 of T-cell and prevents T-cell activation.[5] Efazulimab binds CD11a on surface of T-cell. CD11a is a component of LFA-1. So efazulimab blocks interaction of LFA-1 and ICAM, thereby stopping the inflammatory process.[6]

Etanercept, infliximab and adalimumab inhibit TNF-α activity. Etanercept consists of TNF-α receptor fused with Fc portion of Human IgG.[6] Infliximab is a chimeric (human-mouse) monoclonal antibody acting against human TNF-α. It also causes apoptosis of cells having cell surface TNF-α.[6] Adalimumab is a human recombinant IgG monoclonal antibody with specificity for human TNF-α.[6]

Retinoids effects DNA transcription through binding to RAR (retinoid acid receptor) and RXR (retinoid X receptor). After binding with RARE (retinoid hormone response element) in promoter region of target genes transcription is activated. Target genes that do not contain RARE in promoter region are downregulated by retinoids. This antagonizes transcription factors AP1/NF-IL6, thereby causing anti-proliferative and anti-inflammatory actions.[7]

Calcitriol inhibits proliferation and induces terminal differentiation of keratinocytes. It also increases IL-10 (anti-inflammatory mediator) and decreases IL-8 (pro-inflammatory cytokine).[8]

PHARMACODYNAMICS

The antimitotics are excreted by kidney. Cyclosporine is metabolized by cytochrome P-450 enzyme and excreted in bile and feces.

Side Effects

All the antipsoriatic drugs may increase risk of infections and malignancy. The antimitotics can cause—pancytopenia, mucosal erosions, hepatotoxicity and GIT disturbances. Methotrexate can cause oligospermia.

Alefacept and etanercept can cause reactions in site of injection while efazulimb, infliximab and adalimumab can cause flu-like symptoms. Anemia, leucopenia and thrombocytopenia can be caused by efazulimab. Anti-nuclear antibodies is produced by etanercept, infliximab and adalimumab.

Cyclosporine can cause hypertension, hyperlipemia, headache and tremor when used for short term. Renal interstitial fibrosis develops after 2 years of therapy.

Retinoids can cause teratogenicity; dryness of lips, eyes, skin; DISH (diffuse idiopathic skeletal hyperostoses); increased intracranial tension; dyslipidemia; hepatic toxicity.

Calcitriol can cause hypercalcemia and hypercalciuria.

Contraindications

All drugs are contraindicated in pregnancy, lactation, infections, recent live virus vaccination, immunodeficiency disorders including malignancy, allergy to the particular drug, younger age group, impaired renal function and liver function.

Avoid

Antimitotics and retinoids in—anemia, leucopenia and thrombocytopenia.

Retinoids in—hypercholesterolemia, hypertryglyceridemia, suicidal ideation and pseudotumor cerebri.

Cyclosporine in—hypertension.

Etanercept, infliximab and adalimumab in—multiple sclerosis.

Methotrexate and mycophenolate mofetil in—peptic ulcer.

DRUG INTERACTIONS

Laboratory Investigations

1. CBC (complete blood count)—weekly for 2 weeks; biweekly for 1 month; then monthly. Stop if WBC <3500 cells/mm^3; platelet <125 × 109/L; hemoglobin 110 g/L

2. ESR

3. LFT (liver function test)—monthly for 2 months; then every 4–6 months.

   For methotrexate, liver biopsy after cumulative dose of 1.5 g of methotrexate.

4. RFT (renal function test: serum creatinine, BUN, Na, K, uric acid)—monthly for 2 months; then every 4–6 months. For cyclosporine, RFT done every 2 weeks for 1–2 months; then monthly. Creatinine clearance if >6 months of therapy. Dose is reduced by 25–50% if serum creatinine is elevated by 25% baseline. Stop drug if serum creatinine is elevated by 50% baseline.

5. Urinalysis—every month if abnormal; otherwise yearly.

6. Chest X-ray

7. Pregnancy test

8. Lipid profile for cyclosporine (every 2 weeks for 2 months; then monthly) and retinoids.

DOSAGE

Methotrexate: Test dose of 5–10 mg/week followed 5–6 days later with CBC, RFT and LFT. Gradually increased by 2.5/5 mg every 2–4 weeks until satisfactory results are obtained (max 30 mg/wk). Parenteral administration for patients with erythroderma or who cannot tolerate orally.

Hydroxyurea: 1 to 2g/day (20–30 mg/kg/day) in divided doses.

Thioguanine: 80 mg twice weekly; increase by 20 mg every 2–4 weeks; maximum dose—160 mg 3 times weekly.

Mycophenolate mofetil: Given as 2000–3000 mg daily.

Cyclosporine: Started as 4 mg/kg/day; after clearance or resolution of psoriasis, it should be reduced by 1 mg/kg/day each month and alternate medicine started.

Efazulimab: 1 mg/kg subcutaneously once weekly.

Etanercept: 50 mg twice weekly subcutaneously for 3 months; then 50 mg weekly.

Retinoids: Started at 10 mg/day as initial worsening of the disease occurs; then increased to 25–50 mg/day or 50–75 mg/day.

Calcitriol: 0.5 to 3 µg qhs.

INDICATIONS

Systemic therapy is started if topical therapy and phototherapy is inadequate. It can be given in the following ways:

  i. Monotherapy
 ii. Combination therapy
iii. Rotational therapy
 iv. Sequential therapy

Monotherapy

Monotherapy is the most traditional therapy for psoriasis. First methotrexate, then acitretin and then cyclosporine is started. Of the systemic therapies, acitretin is the least effective as monotherapy and it is therefore often used in conjunction with topical corticosteroid/vitamin D_3/anthralin or UVB or PUVA.

If these drugs fail, treatment with a biologic agent is indicated. Relative and absolute contraindication of each drug is considered before starting treatment. Methotrexate is contraindicated in patients with excessive alcohol intake or active hepatitis. Cyclosporine is contraindicated in patients with hypertension or renal insufficiency.

When remission occurs, methotrexate, acitretin or fumarates can be used as maintenance therapy.

Monotherapy has the advantages of lower cost and greater adherence by the patient. Monotherapy can result in loss of efficacy, adverse effects, cumulative or acute toxicity and inability to clear resistant lesions. Combination, rotational, and sequential approaches are often more effective and safer than monotherapy.[9]

Combination Therapy

When a single drug does not provide remission, they can be used in combination. Combinations of each drug with topical agents (retinoids, steroids, vitamin D derivatives, and others) are beneficial. Combining calcipotriol with cyclosporin or acitretin reduces the dose of cyclosporin or acetretin. Hydroxyurea, thioguanine and biologic agents, have also shown some success in combination therapy. Combination of cyclosporine with acitretin or methotrexate is contraindicated because of increased accumulation of cyclosporine or cutaneous malignancies respectively.[9]

Rotational Therapy

Rotational therapy relies on the concept that even if a patient is doing well, you should rotate from one treatment to another so that the cumulative long-term side effects of any one agent can be avoided. Rotational therapy is mainly applicable for methotrexate, which has a cumulative effect on the liver, or cyclosporine, which has a cumulative effect on the kidneys. It is not as important for the biologic agents, some of which do not seem to have cumulative long-term side effects.[10]

Sequential Therapy

Sequential therapy involves the use of specific therapeutic agents in a sequence to optimize the therapeutic outcome. Sequential therapy involves 3 main steps: (1) the clearing phase; (2) the transitional phase; and (3) the maintenance phase. An acute exacerbation of psoriasis is treated with cyclosporine at a dose of 5 mg/kg daily. After 1 month, the transitional phase is initiated with the gradual introduction of acitretin as a maintenance agent. Once the maximum tolerated dose of acitretin has been established, cyclosporine is gradually tapered and acitretin is continued for long-term maintenance. Phototherapy (UVB or PUVA) is added for improved control if needed.

REFERENCES

1. Gudjonsson JE, Elder JT. Psoriasis. In:Goldsmith LA, Katz SI et al. (eds). Fitzpatrick's dermatology in general medicine. New York: McGraw Hill, 2012, pp197–231

2. Olsen EA. The mechanism of action of methotrexate. Rheum Dis Clin North Am 1997;23:739–55.

3. McDonald CJ. Cytotoxic agents for use in dermatology. J Am Acad Dermatol 1985;12:753–75.

4. Nunley JR, Wolverton S, et al. Systemic drugs. In: Bolognia JL, Jorizzo JL et al (Eds). Dermatology. Spain: Mosby Elsevier, 2008, pp2005–20.

5. Chabner BA, Amrein PC, et al. Antineoplastic agents. In: Bruton LL, Lazo JS, Parker KL (Eds). Goodman and Gilman's the pharmacological basis of therapeutics. New York: McGraw-Hill, 2006, pp1335–39.

6. Callen JP. Immunomodulators. In: Bolognia JL, Jorizzo JL, et al. (Eds). Dermatology. Spain: Mosby Elsevier, 2008, pp1973–90.

7. Kuenzli S, Saurat JH. Retinoids. In: Bolognia JL, Jorizzo JL, et al. (Eds). Dermatology. Spain: Mosby Elsevier, 2008, pp1935–48.

8. Fukuoka M, Ogino Y, Sato H, et al. RANTES expression in psoriatic skin, and regulation of RANTES and IL-8 production in cultured epidermal keratinocytes by active vitamin D_3 (tacalcitol). Br J Dermatol 1998;138: 63–70.

9. Lebwohl M, Menter A, Koo J, Feldman SR. Combination therapy to treat moderate to severe psoriasis.

10. Van de Kerkhof PC. Therapeutic strategies: Rotational therapy and combinations. Clin Exp Dermatol 2001 Jun;26(4):356–61.

13

Systemic Drug in Psoriasis

Vidya Kharkar

INTRODUCTION

Numerous topical and systemic therapies are available for the treatment of the cutaneous manifestations of psoriasis. Treatment modalities are chosen on the basis of disease severity, relevant comorbidities, patient preference (including cost and convenience), efficacy, and evaluation of individual patient response. Although medication safety plays an important role in treatment selection, this must be balanced by the risk of under treatment of psoriasis, leading to inadequate clinical improvement and patient dissatisfaction.

American Academy of Dermatology published guidelines for the management of psoriasis with systemic therapies.

Options for systemic therapy include immunosuppressive or immunomodulatory drugs such as methotrexate, cyclosporine, and biologic agents. Systemic retinoids, which improve psoriasis through effects on epidermal proliferation and differentiation as well as immunomodulation, are also used for the treatment of this condition. Also narrowband UV-B, PUVA, and excimer laser are used for treating psoriasis.

In this chapter we will be discussing only the common drugs used in the treatment of psoriasis, like methotrexate, cyclosporine, and acitretin. Phototherapy and biological effects have been discussed separately.

METHOTREXATE

Methotrexate (MTX) is a folic acid antagonist, used successfully in the treatment of psoriasis for over 30 years. It is also effective for the treatment of psoriatic arthritis and psoriatic nail disease.

Mechanism of Action

The mechanism of action, initially was centered around the anti-proliferative effects of methotrexate on DNA synthesis in epidermal cells; subsequent evidence supports the concept that it is the immunosuppressive effects of methotrexate on activated T-cells that controls psoriasis.

MTX has activity as an immunosuppressive agent. The effect probably occurs because of inhibition of DNA synthesis in immunologically competent cells. The drug can suppress primary and secondary antibody responses.There is no significant effect on delayed-type hypersensitivity.

Indications

Indications for methotrexate therapy of psoriasis:
- Erythrodermic psoriasis
- Psoriatic arthritis: Not responsive to conventional therapy
- Pustular psoriasis: Generalized or debilitating localized disease
- Psoriasis that adversely affects ability to maintain employment
- Extensive, severe plaque psoriasis: Not responsive to conventional therapy (usually >20% surface involvement)
- Lack of response to phototherapy (PUVA and UVB) or systemic retinoids

Pre-treatment workup:
- History and clinical examination
- Objective assessment of the disease (such as PASI)
- HRQoL (Health related quality of life)
- Laboratory parameters
- Chest X-ray
- Contraception in women of child-bearing age (starting after menstruation), and also in men
- If abnormalities in liver screening are found, refer patient to specialist for further evaluation

During treatment:
- Objective assessment of the disease (such as PASI)
- HRQoL (health related quality of life)
- Check concomitant medication
- Clinical examination
- Laboratory controls
- Contraception in women of child-bearing age, and also in men
- 5 mg folic acid once weekly 24 hours after MTX

Post-treatment:
- Women must not become pregnant and men must not be the father of the child for at least three months

Adverse Drug Reactions/Safety

The prevalence and severity of side effects depend on the dose and dosing regimen. If AEs occur, the dose should be decreased or the therapy discontinued, and reconstructive measures instituted, such as supplementation with folic acid. The two most important ADR associated with MTX therapy are myelo-suppression and hepatotoxicity.

The assessment of the risk of severe liver damage from MTX and the recommendations for screening differ. They range from regular serum liver function tests to liver biopsy according to certain time and dose intervals. Liver biopsy has been the standard for detecting liver fibrosis and cirrhosis. Today, however, most European countries have adopted the alternative of assaying procollagen type-III N-terminal peptide (PIIINP) in serum.

Most causes of death due to MTX are the result of bone marrow suppression. Informing patients about the early symptoms of pancytopenia (dry cough, nausea, fever, dyspnoea, cyanosis, stomatitis/oral symptoms, and bleeding) may aid early detection. Hypoalbuminemia and reduced renal function increase the risk of ADR. Special care should be taken when treating geriatric patients, in whom doses should usually be lower and kidney function monitored regularly.

Overview of Important Side Effects

Very frequent
- Nausea, malaise, hair loss

Frequent
- Elevated transaminases, bone marrow suppression, gastrointestinal ulcers

Occasional
- Fever, chills, depression, infections

Rare
- Nephrotoxicity, liver fibrosis, and cirrhosis

Very rare
- Interstitial pneumonia, alveolitis

Risk Factors for Liver Disease

Primary
- History of or current excessive alcohol abuse
- Abnormal liver function test
- History of liver disease, including chronic hepatitis

Secondary
- Diabetes mellitus
- Obesity
- Exposure to hepatotoxic drugs or chemicals

Important Contraindications/Restrictions on Use

Absolute contraindications
- Severe infections
- Severe liver disease
- Renal failure
- Conception (men and women)/breastfeeding
- Alcohol abuse
- Bone marrow dysfunction/hematologic changes
- Immunodeficiency
- Acute peptic ulcer
- Significantly reduced lung function

Relative Contraindications
- Kidney or liver disorders
- Old age
- Ulcerative colitis
- History of hepatitis
- Lack of compliance
- Active desire to have a child for women of childbearing age and men
- Gastritis
- Diabetes mellitus
- Previous malignancies
- Congestive heart failure

Therapeutic Recommendations
- MTX is recommend for the induction and long-term treatment.
- MTX can be given by oral or subcutaneous delivery.

Dosing

- Consider test dose: 2.5 to 5.0 mg
- Average dose: 10 to 15 mg/week
- Maximum dose: 30 mg/week
- Upon improvement, taper by 2.5 mg every four weeks
  As recommended by "The National Psoriasis Foundation".

MTX in Different Dosages

MTX 15 mg compared to MTX 7.5 mg

No difference was found between MTX 15 mg and MTX 7.5 mg based on absolute PASI reduction (very low quality).

MTX 25 mg vs MTX 10 mg

MTX 25 mg is superior to MTX 10 mg in the induction therapy based on final PASI score (low quality) and PGA 'clear' (moderate quality) but no difference was seen for PASI 75 (low quality). The high dosage shows a slightly faster onset of action than the low dosage (very low quality).

Overdose/Measures in Case of Overdose

In MTX overdose, clinical manifestations of acute toxicity include myelosuppression, mucosal ulceration (particularly of the oral mucosa), and rarely, cutaneous necrolysis. The last of these complications is also occasionally seen in patients with very active, extensive psoriasis when the dose of MTX is increased too rapidly. Relative overdose is usually precipitated by factors that interfere with MTX renal excretion or by drug interactions.

Measures in case of overdose: Administer folinic acid (calcium leucovorin) immediately at 20 mg (or 10 mg/m^2) intravenously or intramuscularly. Subsequent doses should be given at six-hour intervals either parenterally or orally.

Management Options

Side effects requiring therapy.

Management Tips

Nausea

- 5 mg folic acid; do not give on day of MTX treatment due to possible reduction in efficacy

- Decrease or divide MTX dose
- Administer SQ or IM

Aphthous Stomatitis

Check CBC

- Dose related and reversible—lower dose
- Add topical treatment
- Folic acid, although it may reduce the efficacy
- Leucovorin—do not give on the day MTX is given

Increased LFTs

- Check LFTs 5–7 days after dose—(WHO guidelines for liver toxicity).

WHO Guidelines for liver toxicity

- Grade 0 toxicity (none)—ALT/AST <1.25x normal
- Grade 1 (mild)—ALT/AST 1.26–2.5x normal; re-check in 2–4 weeks
- Grade 2 (moderate)—ALT/AST 2.6–5x normal; lower MTX dose
- Grade 3 (severe)—ALT/AST 5.1–10x normal; stop MTX and re-check in 2 weeks
- Grade 4 (life threatening)—ALT/AST >10x normal; stop MTX, life threatening
  - Ask about alcohol, medicines such as acetaminophen, ASA
  - Increased GGT and alkaline phosphatase not related to MTX
  - Consider liver biopsy (liver biopsy findings)

AST (SGOT)/ALT (SGPT)

Liver biopsy findings

- *Grade I (normal; mild fatty infiltration, nuclear variability, portal hypertension)*
  - Continue MTX
- *Grade II (moderate and severe; fatty infiltration, nuclear variability, portal tract inflammation)*
  - Continue MTX
- *Grade IIIA (mild fibrosis)*
  - May continue MTX; repeat biopsy in 6 months

Grade IIIB (moderate and severe fibrosis)
- Discontinue MTX

Grade IV (cirrhosis)
- Discontinue MTX

Bone marrow suppression (decreased Hct, megaloblastic anemia)
- Monitor for drug interaction with NSAIDs, trimethorprim/ sulphamethoxazole
- Lower MTX dose if symptomatic
- Folate, 5 mg/day

Platelets
- Any sudden and/or significant reduction in platelet count from pre-treatment level, repeat CBC and platelet count in 1 week and consider reducing dose

Platelets <normal
- Considering lowering dose and repeat platelet count more often

Platelets 100,000 to normal
- Reduce dose or discontinue MTX

Platelets <100,000
- Discontinue MTX

Side Effects Requiring Therapy
Management tips

WBC
WBC < normal
- Consider lowering dose and repeat WBC more often

WBC 3000 to normal
- Reduce dose or discontinue MTX

WBC < 3000
- Discontinue MTX

Pulmonary Toxicity—Acute Pneumonitis
- Monitor for cough
- Stop MTX; do chest X-ray immediately

Pregnancy/Reproduction Contraindicated
- Men and women must be off MTX for 3 months before conception
- If women becomes pregnant during therapy, discontinue MTX
- If partner of man on MTX becomes pregnant, man stays on MTX, uses condoms, gets genetic counseling

Drug Interactions

Clinical Pearls Regarding MTX

Give patients the risks of methotrexate in writing. The National Psoriasis Foundation brochure on systemic treatments is a convenient, free resource in this regard *www.psoriasis.org/severe/systemics*

- Do not discontinue MTX abruptly, unless doing so is essential.
- Consider supplementing MTX treatment with 1–5 mg daily of folic acid (folate), regardless of whether the patient is experiencing nausea or other gastrointestinal (GI) adverse effects.
- Drug interactions are numerous.

List of most important drugs with potential interactions drug	*Type of interaction*
Colchicines, CSA, NSAID, penicillin, probenecid, salicylates, sulfonamides	Decreased renal elimination of MTX
Chloramphenicol, co-trimoxazole, cytostatic agents, ethanol, NSAID, pyrimethamine, sulfonamides	Increased risk of bone marrow and gastrointestinal toxicity
Barbiturates, co-trimoxazole, phenytoin, probenecid, NSAID, sulfonamides	Interaction with plasma protein binding
ethanol, leflunomide, retinoids, tetracyclines	Increased hepatotoxicity

NSAIDs impair the excretion of MTX, causing bone marrow suppression, but the most lethal combination is MTX with trimethoprim/sulfamethoxazole.

- Use special care when prescribing for the elderly.
- The liquid formulation has a bioavailability similar to that of the tablets and is less expensive, but is more difficult to titrate for elderly patients with poor eyesight.
- Investigations into the use of noninvasive monitoring procedures—such as serologic markers of hepatic fibrosis including serum amino terminal propeptide of type III procollagen (PIIINP)—may help reduce the need for biopsies.

CYCLOSPORINE (Oral Calcineurin Inhibitor) (CSA)

CSA is a highly effective and rapidly acting systemic agent for the treatment of psoriasis. Discovered in 1970 and originally used as an immunosuppressive agent in organ transplantation, it was first shown to be effective for psoriasis in 1979. CSA induces immunosuppression by inhibiting the first phase of T-cell activation. It binds to cyclophillin, with the resulting CSA/cyclophillin complex binding to and inhibiting the enzyme calcineurin, leading to blockade of signal transduction pathways that are dependent on the transcription factor, nuclear factor of activated T cells. This blockade leads to lower levels of multiple inflammatory cytokines including interleukin-2 and interferon gamma, thus inhibiting T-cell activation.

Indications

Psoriasis

There are at least three types of psoriasis that can come under consideration for CSA therapy.

Specific indications for cyclosporine therapy of psoriasis*
- Patients with severe flare-ups
- Patients with severe or disabling psoriasis who cannot tolerate, have contraindications to, or have failed other systemic therapies
- Patient with major life events (such as a wedding) where substantial clearing is critically important

In addition, because CSA is effective for all types of psoriasis, it can be strongly considered for erythrodermic and pustular psoriasis.

CSA is very useful in crisis management, as a bridge to other therapies, and in the rapid treatment of psoriasis unresponsive to other modalities, i.e. as interventional therapy.

Efficacy

CSA given at 2.5 to 5 mg/kg/d for 12 to 16 weeks leads to rapid and dramatic improvement in psoriasis in up to 80% to 90% of patients. When dosed at 3 mg/kg/d, CSA leads to a PASI 75 response in 50% to 70% of patients and a PASI 90 response in 30% to 50% of patients.

Dosage

CSA microemulsion is considered to have a superior pharmacokinetic profile to the regular preparation. CSA should be administered at a consistent time of the day and in relation to meals to decrease the intraindividual blood level variations.

---

*In each of these indications cyclosporine therapy should be given for 3–6 months ideally, 12 months at most.

The CSA solution can be mixed with milk or orange juice but not with grapefruit juice, because this can increase plasma CSA concentrations by inhibiting the cytochrome P450 metabolism of CSA.

To induce remission of psoriasis, the recommended starting dosage of oral cyclosporin is 2.5 mg/kg actual body weight each day, administered in two divided doses.

- If no improvement is evident after 1 month (4 weeks) of 2.5 mg/kg/day, the dosage can be gradually increased in 0.5–1 mg/kg increments, at intervals of 2–4 weeks, up to a maximum of 5 mg/kg/day.
- However, in patients with more severe disease initiate treatment at the highest dosage, when a rapid initial response is required, a starting dosage of 5 mg/kg/day can be used, with stepwise decreases after adequate disease control is achieved.
- Cyclosporine should be stopped if the response is inadequate after 6 weeks administration of 5 mg/kg/day.
- However, after an initially good response, the cyclosporine dosage can be reduced for maintenance therapy in steps of 0.5–1 mg/kg, at intervals of 2 weeks, until the lowest effective dosage level is attained.
- Intermittent cyclosporine therapy may be appropriate for some psoriatic patients, that is, when an initial satisfactory response has been attained, cyclosporine therapy can be stopped and any subsequent relapses treated with reintroduction of cyclosporine at the previously effective dosage.

Pre-treatment workup

- Objective assessment of the disease (such as PASI)
- HRQoL (such as DLQI)
- History and clinical examination should focus on previous and concomitant diseases (e.g. arterial hypertension; severe infections; malignancies, including cutaneous malignancies; renal and liver diseases) and concomitant medication (*see* drug interactions).
- Measurement of the blood pressure on two separate occasions.
- Laboratory controls.
- Reliable contraception (reduced efficacy of progesterone-containing contraceptives).
- Regular gynecologic screening according to national guidelines.
- Consultation on vaccination; susceptibility to infections (take infections seriously, seek medical attention promptly); drug

interactions (inform other treating physicians about therapy); avoidance of excessive sun exposure; use of sunscreens

During Treatment

In uncomplicated long-term therapy with low dose cyclosporine (CSA; 2.5 to 3 mg/kg daily), follow-up intervals may be extended to two months or more. Shorter intervals may be needed in patients with risk factors, dose increases, or those who must take concomitant medications that are likely to contribute to ADR. In selected patients with intermittent and short-term treatment, less strict monitoring (regular checking of blood pressure and creatinine level) may be sufficient.

Objective assessment of the disease (such as PASI)

- HRQoL (such as DLQI)
- Clinical examination should focus on status of skin and mucous membranes (hypertrichosis, gingival changes), signs of infections, gastrointestinal or neurological symptoms (tremor, dysaesthesia), musculoskeletal/joint pain
- Repeat recommendation for sun avoidance and sun protection
- Check of concomitant medication
- Measurement of blood pressure
- Laboratory controls
- Reliable contraception
- Regular gynecologic screening according to national guidelines
- If creatinine is significantly elevated and/or patient on therapy for >1 year, perform creatinine clearance (or creatinine-EDTA clearance where available).
- Determination of the CSA level is recommended in individual cases

Post-treatment

- After discontinuation of CSA, patients should be followed up for skin cancer, especially in case of extensive prior therapeutic or natural UV exposure.

Drug Interactions

Several drug interactions have been documented for cyclosporine, which is extensively metabolised by the CYP 3A system in the liver and small intestine.

- Erythromycin should be used with caution in cyclosporine-treated patients with infected eczema, since the former compound can increase cyclosporine toxicity.
- Grapefruit juice inhibits cyclosporine metabolism and should be avoided in cyclosporine recipients.
- Heavy alcohol ingestion should be avoided, as it can increase cyclosporine levels.
- Nephrotoxic drugs, including aminoglycosides, ciprofloxacin, clotrimazole, fibrates, and nonsteroidal anti-inflammatory drugs (NSAIDs), should not be administered, if at all possible, to cyclosporine-treated patients. NSAIDs, especially in dehydrated patients, are likely to potentiate the deleterious effect of cyclosporine on renal function, and importantly, intermittent NSAID use is often not disclosed by patients.
- Cyclosporine may restrict the metabolism of many drugs (e.g. diclofenac, digoxin, methotrexate, prednisolone, repaglinide, simvastatin), thus increasing plasma levels and toxicity.
- Cyclosporine should not be used concomitantly with potassium-sparing diuretics because of the risk of hyperkalemia, and care should also be exercised if cyclosporine is administered concurrently with potassium-sparing drugs such as angiotensin converting enzyme inhibitors or angiotensin II receptor antagonists.

Important Side Effects

Frequent	Renal failure (dose-dependent); danger of irreversible renal damage (long-term therapy); hypertension; gingival hyperplasia; reversible hepatogastric complaints (dose dependent); tremor; weariness; headache; burning sensation in hands and feet; reversible elevated blood lipids (especially in combination with corticosteroids); hypertrichosis
Occasional	Seizures, gastrointestinal ulcerations, weight gain, hyperglycemia, hyperuricemia, hyperkalemia, hypomagnesemia, acne, anemia
Rare	Ischemic heart disease, pancreatitis, motor polyneuropathy, impaired vision, defective hearing, central ataxia, myopathy, erythema, itching, leucopoenia, thrombocytopenia
Very rare	Microangiopathic hemolytic anemia, hemolytic uremic syndrome, colitis (isolated cases), papillary

edema (isolated cases), idiopathic intracranial hypertension (isolated cases)

Malignancy risk: The risk of non-melanoma skin cancer (NMSC) is probably increased in those patients with psoriasis who are undergoing long-term treatment with CSA.

The incidence of skin cancer, most of which were squamous cell carcinoma, was 6 times higher in psoriasis patients treated with CSA than in the general population. Patients treated for more than 2 years with CSA were shown to have a higher risk. It is not known how much CSA contributes to the risk of skin cancer, as the patients were often exposed to carcinogens (e.g. PUVA) known to cause skin cancers.

When CSA is used in the following fashion, the risk of internal malignancy has yet to be convincingly shown to be increased:

1. Maximum 'dermatologic' dose of 5 mg/kg daily;
2. Continuous therapy for less than 2 years at a time;
3. In psoriasis patients who do not take other systemic immuno-suppressants concurrently; and
4. In psoriasis patients who are generally healthy.

Important contraindications/restrictions on use

Absolute contraindications

- Impaired renal function
- Insufficiently controlled arterial hypertension
- Severe infectious disease
- History of malignancy (possible exceptions: treated basal cell carcinoma, history of squamous carcinoma *in situ*)
- Current malignancy
- Simultaneous PUVA therapy

Relative contraindications

- Previous potential carcinogenic therapies (e.g. arsenic, PUVA >1000 J/cm^2)
- Psoriasis triggered by severe infection or drugs (beta-blockers, lithium, anti-malarial drugs)
- Significant hepatic diseases
- Hyperuricemia
- Hyperkalemia
- Simultaneous therapy with nephrotoxic drugs (*see* drug inter-actions)

- Simultaneous phototherapy
- Simultaneous use of other systemic immunosuppressive agents
- Simultaneous use of systemic retinoids or therapy with retinoids in the last four weeks prior to planned onset of therapy with CSA
- Drug or alcohol-related diseases
- Long-term previous treatment with MTX
- Pregnancy/breastfeeding

Vaccination with live vaccines
- Epilepsy

ACITRETIN

Acitretin is an effective treatment for psoriasis. A major problem with systemic retinoids is their teratogenicity, making contraception mandatory in women of childbearing age during treatment.

Indications

- Severe psoriasis that cannot be managed by topical treatments or photo(chemo) therapy
- Monotherapy is indicated for erythrodermic or pustular psoriasis
- Combination therapy is indicated for chronic plaque psoriasis

Contraindications

- Severe liver dysfunction*
- Severe kidney dysfunction (elimination reduced)*
- Pregnancy or lactation*
- Women of childbearing potential who cannot guarantee adequate contraception during and up to 3 years following discontinuation of acitretin.*
- Hyperlipidemia, especially hypertriglyceridemia, that cannot be controlled.*
- Concomitant medications that interfere with retinoid bio-availability or whose metabolism is altered.[†]
- Concomitant hepatotoxic drugs, e.g. methotrexate[‡]

---

[*]Absolute contraindications.

[†]Requires dose adjustment and careful monitoring, e.g. phenytoin competes for plasma protein binding.

[‡]Reserved for treatment-resistant patients.

- Poorly controlled diabetes mellitus
- History of pancreatitis
- Excessive alcohol intake*
- Use of contact lenses
- Unreliable patient*
- Atherosclerosis

Blood donation is contraindicated in patients receiving acitretin.

Dose

In patients with chronic plaque psoriasis, 0.5 mg/kg/day is the initial dosage, which can be increased depending upon the clinical response and side effects.

For erythrodermic psoriasis, the initial dosage is 0.25 mg/kg/day.

In pustular psoriasis, the dose should be maximized, i.e. doses up to 1 mg/kg/day.

In patients with chronic plaque psoriasis, mild cheilitis (just perceived by the patient) is the goal, whereas in patients with pustular psoriasis, a dose that causes a clinically apparent but tolerable cheilitis is an endpoint.

The efficacy of acitretin monotherapy in chronic plaque psoriasis is limited.

Many of the plaques may remain, but they are thinner with less scale and erythema. 20% of patients may be considered treatment failures.

The efficacy of low-dose acitretin at 10 mg/day was not significantly different from that of placebo in two studies.

Acitretin has been shown to be an effective maintenance therapy. As monotherapy, acitretin is highly effective in erythrodermic and pustular psoriasis. Its efficacy in nail psoriasis and psoriatic arthritis is only modest.

Pre-acitretin Screening

- History to exclude contraindications
- Complete blood count
- Liver function tests (AST, ALT, γ-GT, alkaline phosphatase, bilirubin)

---

*Absolute contraindications.

- Serum triglycerides, cholesterol, HDL
- Glucose
- Serum creatinine
- Pregnancy test
- Consider spinal X-ray (often initially performed during the first 3 months of therapy if long-term treatment is anticipated).

(Pre-acitretin screening. ALT, alanine aminotransferase; AST, aspartate aminotransferase; γ-GT, γ-glutamyl transpeptidase; HDL, high-density lipoproteins).

Evaluation during Acitretin Treatment

- Monitor mucocutaneous side effects
- Serum cholesterol/triglycerides/HDL and liver enzymes (every month for the first 2 months then every 2–3 months)
- Serum creatinine (elderly patients or patients with mild to moderate renal dysfunction)
- Monitor for development of hyperostosis by history (twice yearly) and by X-ray of spine (e.g. once yearly in patients receiving long-term treatment)
- Pregnancy test (throughout treatment)

Overview of important side effects of Acitretin

Very frequent	Vitamin A toxicity (xerosis, cheilitis)
Frequent	Conjunctival inflammation (contact lenses), hair loss, photosensitivity, hyperlipidemia
Occasional	Muscle, joint, and bone pain, retinoid dermatitis
Rare	Gastrointestinal complaints, hepatitis, jaundice, bone changes with long-term therapy
Very rare	Idiopathic intracranial hypertension, decreased color vision and impaired night vision

List of most important drugs with potential interactions

Drug	Type of interaction
Methotrexate	Liver toxicity
Tetracycline	Induction of idiopathic intracranial hypertension
Phenytoin	Plasma protein displacement
Vitamin A	Augmentation of retinoid effect

Low-dose progesterone pills   Insufficient contraceptive effect
Lipid-lowering drugs   Increased risk of myotoxicity
Antifungal imidazoles   Liver toxicity

Concurrent use of retinoids with alcohol may increase conversion of acitretin to etretinate and hepatotoxicity.

Safety

Several potential adverse effects have been associated with acitretin but these can generally be minimized by appropriate patient selection, careful dosing, and monitoring.

Teratogenicity is the most important safety issue. Acitretin is FDA pregnancy category X (highly unsafe during pregnancy, with the risk of use outweighing any possible benefit). The use of any dose of acitretin during pregnancy may lead to numerous malformations, including cardiovascular, ocular, auditory, central nervous system, craniofacial, and skeletal, with the greatest risk occurring between the third and sixth weeks of gestation. Acitretin is contraindicated in women who plan to become pregnant or who fail to use adequate contraception for 3 years after discontinuing acitretin. Under almost every circumstance, acitretin should not be used in women of childbearing potential.

RECOMMENDED READING

1. Armstrong AW, Robertson AD, Wu J, et al. Undertreatment, treatment trends, and treatment dissatisfaction among patients with psoriasis and psoriatic arthritis in the United States: Findings from the National Psoriasis Foundation surveys, 2003–2011. JAMA Dermatol 2013; 149:1180.

2. Berth-Jones J, Henderson CA, Munro CS, Rogers S, Chalmers RJ, Boffa MJ, et al. Treatment of psoriasis with intermittent short course cyclosporin (Neoral): A multicenter study. Br J Dermatol 1997;136: 527–30.

3. Cyclosporine Tina Bhutani, Chai Sue Lee, John YM Koo. In Comprehensive Dermatologic Drug Therapy Stephen E. Wolverton MD, Theodore Arlook Professor of Clinical Dermatology, Department of Dermatology Indiana University School of Medicine; Chief of Dermatology Roudebush VA Medical Center Indianapolis, In, USA 3rd edn, Saunders is an imprint of Elsevier Inc. Edinburgh, 2013;205.

4. Dogra S, Krishna V, Kanwar AJ. Efficacy and safety of systemic methotrexate in two fixed doses of 10 mg or 25 mg orally once weekly

in adult patients with severe plaque-type psoriasis: A prospective, randomized, double-blind, dose-ranging study. Clin Exp Dermatol 2012;37(7):729–34.

5. Faerber L, Braeutigam M, Weidinger G, Mrowietz U, Christophers E, Schulze HJ, et al. Cyclosporine in severe psoriasis: results of a meta-analysis in 579 patients. Am J ClinDermatol 2001;2:41–7.

6. Goldfarb MT, Ellis CN, Gupta AK, et al: Acitretin improves psoriasis in a dose-dependent fashion. J Am Acad Dermatol 1988;18:655–62.

7. Gollnick H, Bauer R, Brindley C, et al. Acitretin versus etretinate in psoriasis. Clinical and pharmacokinetic results of a German multicenter study. J Am Acad Dermatol 1988;19:458–69.

8. Ho VC, Griffiths CE, Albrecht G, Vanaclocha F, Leon-Dorantes G, Atakan N, et al. Intermittent short courses of cyclosporine (Neoral(R)) for psoriasis unresponsive to topical therapy: A 1-year multicenter, randomized study; the PISCES study group. Br J Dermatol 1999;141: 283–91.

9. Ho VC, Griffiths CE, Berth-Jones J, Papp KA, Vanaclocha F, Dauden E, et al. Intermittent short courses of cyclosporine microemulsion for the long-term management of psoriasis: a 2-year cohort study. J Am Acad Dermatol 2001;44:643–51.

10. Lassus A, Geiger JM, Nyblom M, et al. Treatment of severe psoriasis with etretin (Ro 10-1670). Br J Dermatol 1987;117:333–41.

11. Laurie Barclay, Updated Guidelines Address Management of Plaque Psoriasis Arch Dermatol 2012;148:95–102.

12. Lebwohl M. Acitretin in combination with UVB or PUVA. J Am Acad Dermatol 1999;41:S22–S24.

13. Maybury CM, Jabbar-Lopez ZK, Wong T, Dhillon AP, Barker JN, Smith CH. Methotrexate and liver fibrosis in people with psoriasis: a systematic review of observational studies. Br J Dermatol 2014;171(1):17–29.

14. Maybury CM, Samarasekera E, Douiri A, Barker JN, Smith CH. Diagnostic accuracy of noninvasive markers of liver fibrosis in patients with psoriasis taking methotrexate: a systematic review and meta-analysis. Br J Dermatol 2014;170(6):1237–47.

15. Menter A, Gottlieb A, Feldman SR, et al. Guidelines of care for the management of psoriasis and psoriatic arthritis: Section 1. Overview of psoriasis and guidelines of care for the treatment of psoriasis with biologics. J Am Acad Dermatol 2008;58:826.

16. Menter A, Griffiths CE. Current and future management of psoriasis. Lancet 2007;370:272.

17. Menter A, Korman NJ, Elmets CA, et al. Guidelines of care for the management of psoriasis and psoriatic arthritis: section 4. Guidelines of care for the management and treatment of psoriasis with traditional systemic agents. J Am Acad Dermatol 2009;61:451.

18. Methotrexate Jeffrey P. Callen and Carol L. Kulp-Shorten In: Comprehensive Dermatologic Drug Therapy Stephen E. Wolverton MD, Theodore Arlook Professor of Clinical Dermatology, Department of Dermatology, Indiana University School of Medicine; Chief of Dermatology Roudebush VA Medical Center Indianapolis, In: USA 3rd edn, Saunders is an imprint of Elsevier Inc. Edinburgh, 2013;171.

19. Mueller W, Herrmann B. Cyclosporin A for psoriasis. N Engl J Med 1979;301:555.

20. Pathirana D, et al. JEADV. 2009; 23 (Suppl 2):1–69.

21. Prens EP, van Joost T, Hegmans JP, 9tHooft-Benne K, Ysselmuiden OE, Benner R. Effects of cyclosporine on cytokines and cytokine receptors in psoriasis. J Am Acad Dermatol 1995;33:947–53.

22. Strober BE, Siu K, Menon K. Conventional systemic agents for psoriasis. A systematic review. J Rheumatol 2006;33:1442.

14

Phototherapy in Psoriasis

Sathish Pai B

INTRODUCTION

Phototherapy is one of the most useful and effective treatment options in the management of psoriasis vulgaris. Neils Ryberg Finsen is the father of modern phototherapy. He was the first person to develop artificial source of radiation in the treatment of lupus vulgaris for which he received Nobel Prize in the year 1903.[1] Psoralen photochemotherapy (PUVA) was found to be effective in the treatment of psoriasis in the mid-1970s and fluorescent tubes emitting a narrow spectrum of UVB rays in the range of 311 to 313 were discovered in the mid-1980s and were found to be beneficial in psoriasis.[2] This discovery is referred to as Narrow Band UVB phototherapy (NBUVB). Phototherapy is indicated when psoriasis involves more than 10% of the body surface area[1] but can be used in patients with severe scalp and palmoplantar psoriasis, where the involvement is less than 5%. Limited disease over these areas can affect the quality of life of the patient. The primary goal of treating psoriasis is to clear the disease and keep it under control.

TYPES OF PHOTOTHERAPY

Phototherapy in psoriasis is basically of two types; PUVA and NBUVB.

INDICATIONS FOR PHOTOTHERAPY

1. Moderate to severe psoriasis
2. Failure of topical therapy
3. When systemic drugs are contraindicated or poorly tolerated

PSORALEN PHOTOCHEMOTHERAPY (PUVA)

Here the drug psoralen is used along with long wave ultraviolet radiation (UVA) (320 to 400 nm). Commonly available psoralens are 8-methoxypsoralen (8-MOP) and trimethlypsoralen (TMP). 8-MOP is obtained from plants, whereas trimethylpsoralen is a synthetic psoralen.

Psoralens can be used orally or in bath water for the treatment of psoriasis. The drug psoralen sensitizes the cells to the effect of ultraviolet A radiation. The therapeutic effect is seen only when the two are combined. PUVA is responsible for inducing a well regulated repetitive phototoxic reaction, which does not occur if either of it is used solely.

Mechanism of Action of PUVA in Psoriasis[3]

1. Inhibition of cell proliferation
2. Immunomodulatory action

Inhibition of Cell Proliferation

The psoralen molecule first enters the cell and intercalates between the nucleic acid bases. When the skin is exposed to UVA radiation, it absorbs a photon form the ultraviolet A radiation and gets excited. The excited psoralen covalently binds to pyrimidine base and forms a photoproduct or photoadduct. This photoadduct absorbs another photon and causes linking of psoralen molecule to pyrimidine base on opposite DNA strand thus cross-linking the two DNA strand (Fig. 14.1). These cross-links are toxic to the cell and inhibit DNA synthesis and thus the cell proliferation. PUVA also inhibits the mTOR signaling pathway which regulates the cell growth and proliferation.[3]

Immunomodulatory Action

PUVA has got various immunomodulatory actions. It causes apoptosis of lymphocytes, alters the function of antigen presenting cells and alters the cytokine profile. In psoriasis the helper T cells get activated and convert to form Th1 and Th17 cells, which release various cytokines that cause inflammation and hyperproliferation of cells.[4] PUVA inhibits Th1 and Th17 pathways and stimulates Th2 cells with the release of cytokines like IL-10 and IL-4 which brings about improvement in psoriasis.

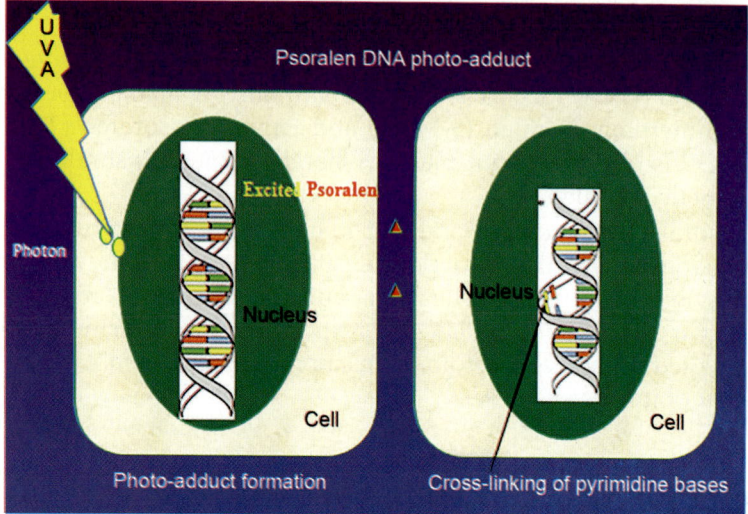

Fig. 14.1 Formation of psoralen-DNA photo-adduct and cross-linking of pyrimidine bases

Methods of Administration of PUVA

1. Oral PUVA
2. Oral PUVASOL
3. Bath water PUVA
4. Bathing suit PUVA

Oral PUVA

Oral 8-methoxypsoralen (8-MOP) is given in the dose of 0.6 to 0.8 mg/kg body weight one and half to two hours before administering UVA in a whole body phototherapy chamber. Since it is difficult to determine the minimal phototoxic dose (MPD) on Indian skin, the UVA dose is based on the skin type. The initial starting dose of UVA for Indian skin is usually between 2 and 3 J/sq cm^5 with increments of 0.5 J/sq. cm. The increments are given if there is no erythema or burning of the skin. The treatment is given two to three times per week till clearance. Normally psoriasis clears after 20 to 25 treatments. Once there is clearance the dose of UVA is kept constant and frequency of treatment is gradually reduced to once weekly, then once in two weeks and then to as low as once in a month. The maintenance phase is given for 2 to 3 months and the treatment is then stopped.

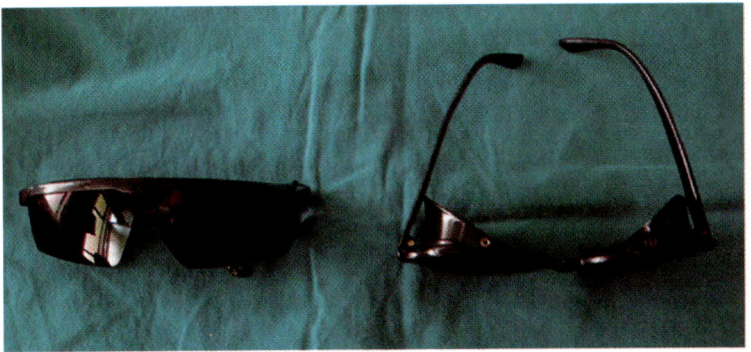

Fig. 14.2 B2 Toric glasses for eye protection

Precautions for oral PUVA

1. The eyes should be protected with UVA protective glasses like B2 Toric (Fig. 14.2) or green 60 while administering UVA and also on the days when oral psoralens are taken if the patient is going out in the sun.
2. Patients should avoid exposing their skin to direct sunlight on the days of PUVA treatment. A suitable sunscreen should be used to protect the skin from the harmful effects of sunlight on days of PUVA treatment.
3. Patients should avoid perfumes, deodorants and aftershave lotion on days of PUVA treatment.

Contraindications for PUVA

1. History of cutaneous malignancy
2. Cardiac insufficiency or inability to stand in the chamber
3. Claustrophobia
4. Immunosuppressed patients
5. Pregnancy
6. Children less than 12 years

Side effects of oral PUVA

1. Erythema
2. Nausea
3. PUVA itch
4. Pigmentation
5. Cataract
6. Skin cancer
7. Photoaging

Oral PUVASOL

Sunlight is the cheapest and easily available source of UVA. When oral psoralen is used along with sunlight as the source of UVA, it is called PUVASOL treatment. PUVASOL therapy is basically indicated in patients who cannot visit the hospital to receive UVA treatment.

Disadvantages of PUVASOL therapy

1. The amount of UVA rays present in the sunlight varies from place to place, time of the day, season and the atmospheric conditions.
2. Other rays present in the sunlight like UVB, infra-red and visible light can produce undesirable side-effects.
3. It is very difficult to estimate the amount of UVA rays present in the sunlight.
4. There is lack of privacy.

When to expose to sunlight

The ideal time to expose to sunlight is between 9.15 AM and 11.15 AM in the morning and 2.30 PM and 3.30 PM in the afternoon.[6] This is the time when incidental rays like UVB and infra-red are relatively less and so is the adverse effects associated with exposure to these rays.

How long to expose to sunlight

The exposure time to sunlight varies from place to place. In a study by Srinivas *et al*[7] it was found that to receive 2J/sq. cm of UVA at 11.00 AM in the month of May 4 minutes of sun exposure was required. The exposure time increases to 6 minutes in the month of December and to 6 minutes 30 seconds in the month of June.

Increments with sun exposure

The sun exposure time can be increased by 1 minute every week which is approximately equivalent to 0.5 J/sq cm. The maximum duration of sun exposure is 30 minutes.

The problem of lack of privacy with PUVASOL therapy can be overcome by using clothes on PUVASOL therapy.[8] A plain woven, cream colored light weight cotton gown (2×2 cotton blouse cloth) (Fig. 14.3) can be worn during sun exposure, but the duration of sun exposure has to be increased by 3.33 times. For example, if the patient has been asked to expose to sunlight for 4 minutes, with the clothes on the exposure time will increase to 13.32 minutes. The problem of privacy can also be overcome by installing a solarium.[9] It consists of a two-room structure which is usually

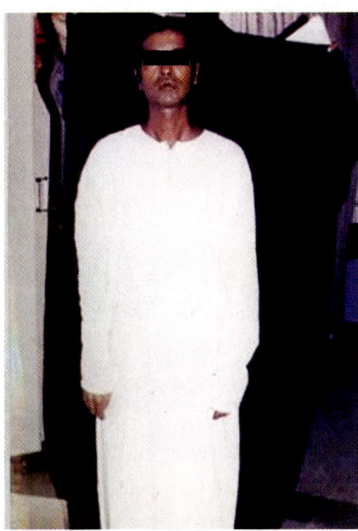

Fig. 14.3 Patient with plain woven cotton gown for clothes on PUVASOL therapy

constructed on the roof top. The roof of the room is made up of 5 mm thick window glass. The window glass blocks UVB rays but allows UVA rays to pass through it. The patient after receiving bath water psoralen or oral psoralen lies down on a raised platform to receive UVA rays from sunlight. The amount of UVA rays present in the sunlight can be measured using a photometer. The only disadvantage of solarium is that the patient has to visit the hospital for therapy.

Bath Water PUVA

Bath PUVA is a very effective treatment for psoriasis.[10] Bath water PUVA gives quick or even quicker response than other systemic therapies in the treatment of psoriasis. The improvement seen may be faster than many of the cytokine antagonist.[10]

Procedure

A bath tub is filled with 100 liters of water. 37.5 ml of 1% 8-methoxy-psoralen is added to 100 liters of water to obtain a concentration of 3.75 mg/liter. A low concentration of 2.6 mg/liter can also be used.[11] The patient then soaks the body for 20 minutes (Fig. 14.4). After 20 minutes of soaking the patient comes out of the tub, gently pat dries the skin and is then immediately exposed to UVA rays in a whole body UVA phototherapy chamber (Fig. 14.5). The eyes

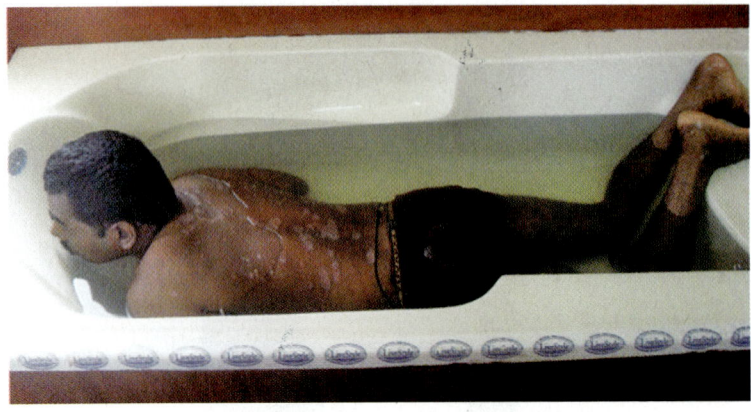

Fig. 14.4 Patient receiving bath water treatment

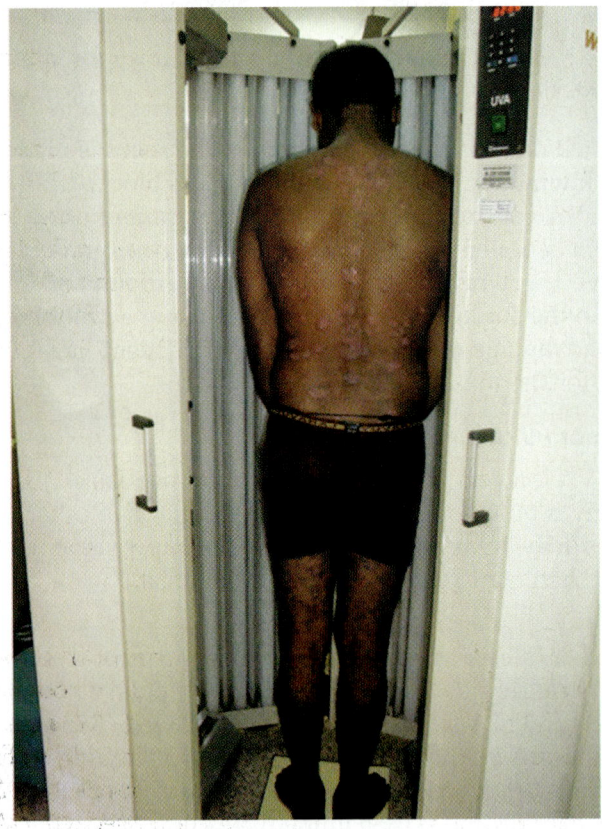

Fig. 14.5 Patient receiving UVA treatment in a whole body UVA chamber

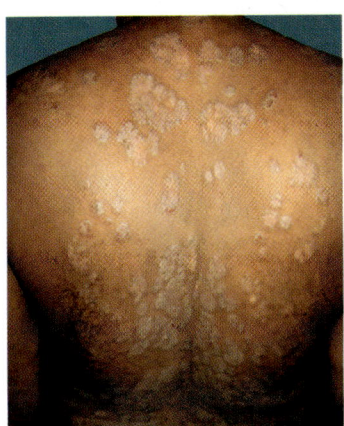

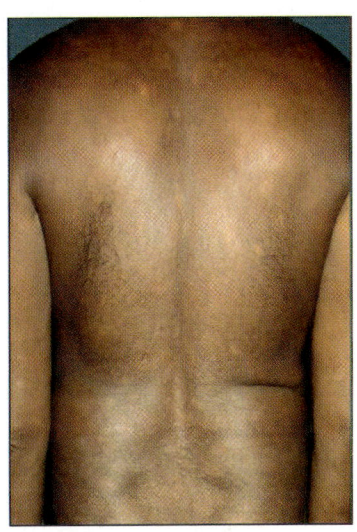

Fig. 14.6 Psoriasis before bath PUVA treatment

Fig. 14.7 Complete clearance of psoriasis after 15 bath PUVA treatments

should be protected with UVA protective goggles and men need to cover their genitalia with dark undergarments.

Treatment is given three times a week. Clearance is usually seen with 12 to 15 treatments (Figs 14.6 and 14.7). After clearance patient is given maintenance therapy for 2 to 3 months. The therapy is given twice weekly initially for a month and then once weekly. If the patient cannot come for maintenance therapy treatment can be stopped after clearance.

UVA protocol
The starting dose of UVA is 0.5 to 1 J/sq. cm with increments of 0.5 J/sq. cm provided there is no erythema or burning sensation.

Side effects
1. Phototoxic reaction[12] (Fig. 14.8)
2. Pruritus[13]
3. Folliculitis[14]
4. Pigmentation[14]

Bathing Suit PUVA[15]

Bathing suit PUVA can be administered in places where bath water facilities are not available and this treatment can also be carried out at home with sunlight as the source of UVA.

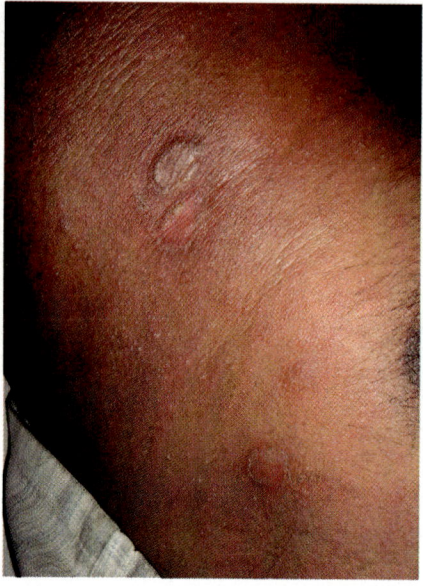

Fig. 14.8 Phototoxic reaction at 72 hours showing diffuse erythema, papules and a few pustules

Procedure

Two liters of water is taken in a bucket. To this 1 ml of 1% 8-methoxypsoralen is added to obtain a concentration of 3.75 mg per liter. A bathing suit made up of flannel material stitched to suit the patient is dipped in the psoralen solution for 5 minutes. After soaking for 5 minutes the suit is removed and is gently squeezed to remove excess water. The patient then wears the suit (Fig. 14.9) for 15 minutes with a rain coat over it to prevent evaporation of water. After 15 minutes the suit is removed and patient is immediately exposed to UVA rays in a whole body UVA phototherapy chamber. Clearance of psoriasis usually occurs after 12–15 treatments (Figs 14.10 and 14.11). The starting dose of UVA is 1 to 2 J/sq cm with increments of 0.5 J/sq cm.

The advantages with bathing suit PUVA are it requires only 2 liters of water and 1 ml of psoralen solution. This therapy can be carried out at home with sunlight as the source of UVA.

PUVA can be combined with various topical and systemic agents. The topical preparations are steroids, calcipotriol, tazarotene, tar and dithranol. Systemically PUVA can be combined with acitretin, methotrexate and NBUVB.

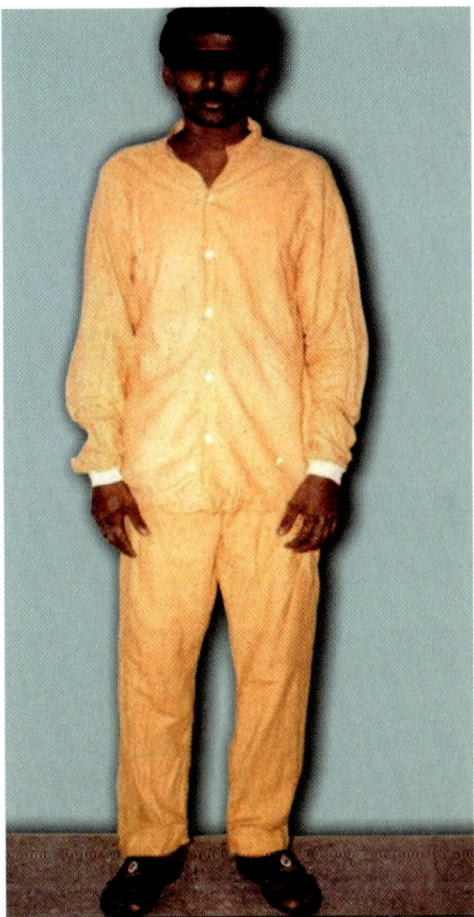

Fig. 14.9 Patient wearing bathing suit for PUVA therapy

Narrowband UVB Phototherapy (NBUVB)

In the year 1978 Wiskeman introduced broad band UVB (BBUVB). The wavelength of broadband ranges from 290 to 320 nm. Fluorescent tubes emitting these rays have been used alone or with crude coal tar in the management of psoriasis. The main drawback of BBUVB rays were that it produced erythema and did not give satisfactory improvement in psoriasis. Narrowband UVB, which emits a narrow spectrum at 311 nm, was found to be effective in the treatment of psoriasis in the year 1988.[16,17] Later it was proved that NBUVB was better than BBUVB in the management of psoriasis.[18]

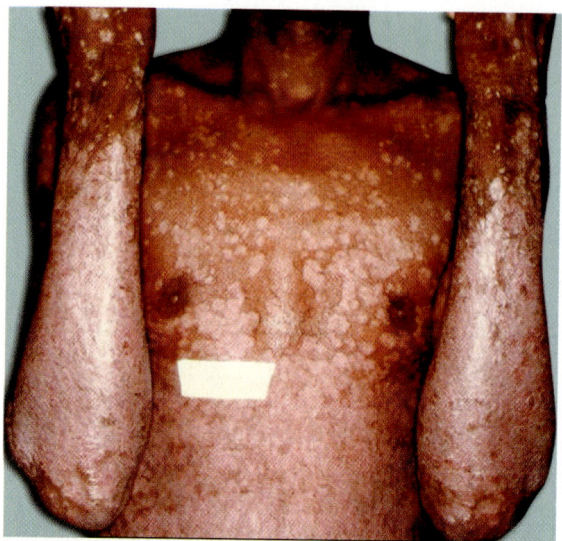

Fig. 14.10 Psoriasis before bathing suit PUVA

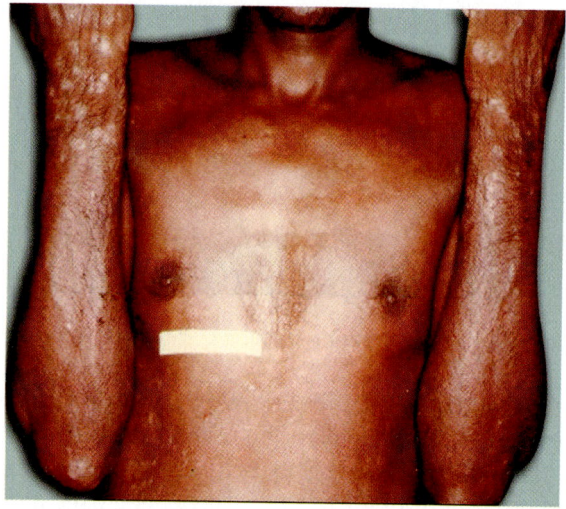

Fig. 14.11 Complete clearance of psoriasis after 15 bathing suit PUVA treatments

Mechanism of Action[19]

1. Direct effect on DNA
2. Release of reactive oxygen species

3. Conversion of *trans*-urocanic acid to *cis*-urocanic acid
4. Apoptosis of T-cells

Direct Action on DNA

UVB radiation produces direct damage to the DNA. It can be absorbed in the epidermis or in the upper dermis as shown in the figure. The rays are absorbed by the thymidine molecules in the DNA. After absorption the molecules get excited undergo a photochemical reaction and form a photoproduct. The photoproduct formed here is a four-membered ring structure called cyclobutane-pyrimidine dimer. These dimers play a pivotal role in producing a beneficial effect and are also important in causing the toxic effects. In psoriasis these dimers inhibit cell proliferation. The dimers also cause mutation, but most of the UV-induced DNA lesions are not converted into mutant cells.

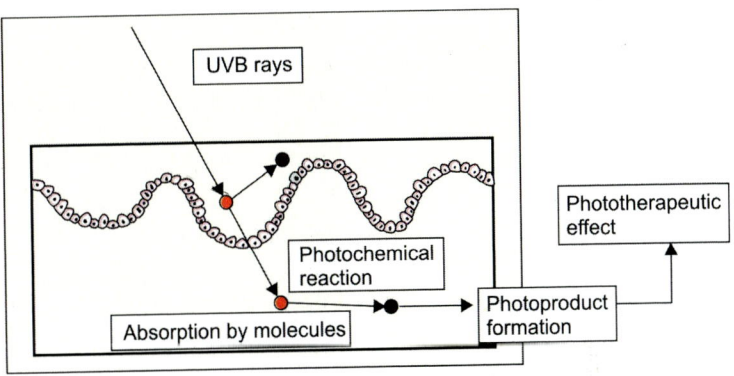

UVB rays generate reactive oxygen species like singlet oxygen, superoxide anion, etc. which leads to release of inflammatory mediators like prostaglandins E2 and cytokines. UVB radiation also isomerizes *trans*-urocanic acid to *cis*-urocanic acid which induces immunosuppression.

NB-UVB is able to inhibit cell proliferation as well as is able to induce apoptosis of various cell types. This action may be responsible for its therapeutic activity in diseases with a high proliferation rate, such as psoriasis.[20]

DOSIMETRY AND TREATMENT PROTOCOL

Minimal erythema dose (MED) determination is advisable in all patients receiving NBUVB phototherapy to ensure optimal dosage schedule for clearance of psoriasis. There are a few and contradictory data on MED on Indian skin.[21–23] When the erythema response to NBUVB varies widely in a population, it is essential to base the starting dose on MED to obtain a satisfactory response to NBUVB phototherapy.[24] Therefore, it would be prudent to estimate the MED in every patient with psoriasis undergoing NBUVB phototherapy to ensure optimal outcome.

MED Determination

A template with 8 windows of 2 sq. cm is made over the back of a cotton suit used by operation theater staff or on a flexible card board. Flaps are made over the windows so that it can be closed and opened whenever required. This template is applied on the back of the patient and other areas are covered with a protective gown (Fig. 14.12). The windows are then exposed to geometric series of NBUVB starting with 300 mj/ sq. cm up to 1080 mj/sq. cm. First all the windows are exposed to 300 mj, then the first window is closed and other windows are exposed to an additional 60 mj, so that the

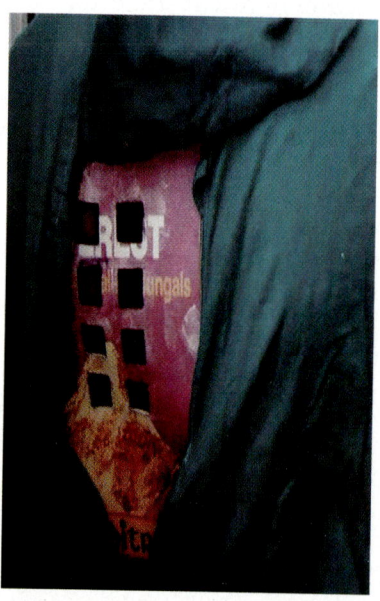

Fig. 14.12 Determination of MED to NBUVB

second window will receive 360 mj. The windows are closed one by one and required doses are delivered. MED is read after 24 hours as just perceptible erythema (Figs 14.13 and 14.14).

Treatment Protocol

In MED-based protocol the starting dose of NBUVB in psoriasis is usually 50 to 70% of MED. The starting dose can also be based on the skin type. As per the US protocol the starting dose of NBUVB for skin type IV and V is 330 mj/sq cm and 350 mj/sq cm respectively.[25] In the European skin type based protocol a higher dose is used, for example, for skin type IV and V a dose of 600 mj/ sq cm and 700 mj/sq cm is used respectiveley.[26]

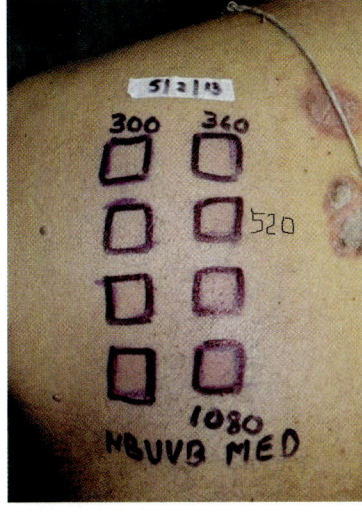

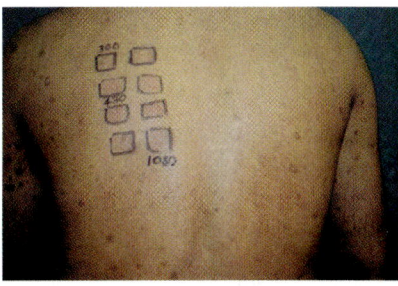

Fig. 14.13 MED seen at 520 mj to NBUVB

Fig. 14.14 MED seen at 430 mj to NBUVB

Increments

Increments are given based on the erythema response as follows:

No erythema: 20% increment

Mild erythema: Previous dose is maintained and subsequent dose increment is reduced to 10%

Moderate erythema: Postpone one treatment, repeat previous dose at the next visit and reduce to 10% increment

Severe erythema: Stop treatment.

The increment schedule may vary depending on the population being treated.

Frequency of Treatment

The current recommendation is three times a week as it is optimal. Phototherapy is given till clearance, i.e. 25 to 30 sittings. Maintenance treatment is normally not recommended for NBUVB phototherapy.

Missed Treatment

If the patient misses treatment for 7 days, then the same dose is given. The dose is reduced by 25 % if treatment is missed for

2 weeks and by 50% if it missed for 3 weeks. It is advisable to restart the treatment if the therapy is missed for more than 3 weeks.

Side Effects

1. Erythema and burning of the skin
2. Pruritus
3. Reactivation of orolabial herpes simplex
4. Exposure keratitis and conjunctivitis
5. Tanning

A systematic review of literature by Archier et al showed that in the management of psoriasis both PUVA and NBUVB were useful treatment modalities, but PUVA gave faster results and longer remission period. They concluded that NBUVB is preferred by treating doctor because of ease of administration.[27]

NBUVB can be combined with topical steroid, calcipotriol, dithranol and tazarotene. Combination of these topical agents gives faster clearance and also reduces the cumulative doses of NBUVB. Systemic agents that can be used along with NBUVB are methotrexate, acitretin and etanercept.

REFERENCES

1. Menter A, Korman NJ, Elmets CA, et al. Guidelines of care for the management of psoriasis and psoriatic arthritis. J Am Acad Dermatol 2010;62:114–35.

2. Honigsmann H, Schwartz T. Ultraviolet therapy. In: Bolognia JL, Jorizzo JL, Rapini RP, Schaffer JV (Eds). Dermatology, 2nd edn. Spain: Mosby; 2008; p.2053.

3. Richard EG, Morison W. Psoralen plus ultraviolet A (PUVA) photochemotherapy. In: UpToDate, Post TW (Ed), UpToDate, Elmets CA. (Accessed on August 15, 2015.)

4. Tami Wong BS, Leon Hsu BA, Wilson Liao MD. Phototherapy in Psoriasis: A Review of Mechanisms of Action. J Cutan Med Surg 2013; 17(1):6–12.

5. Shenoi SD, Prabhu S. Photochemotherapy (PUVA) in psoriasis and vitiligo-therapeutic guidelines. Ind J DermatolVenereolLeprol 2014; 80:497–504.

6. Balasaraswathy P, Kumar U, Srinivas CR, Nair S. UVA and UVB in sunlight. Opitmal utilization of UV rays in sunlight for phototherapy. Indian J Dermatol 2002;68:198–201.

7. Srinivas CR, Devadiga R, Parashar TR, Chandras. Exposure time to sunlight for ultraviolet light therapy. Ind J Dermatol Venereol Leprol 1989;57:17–18.

8. Varma S, Ballambat SP, Balachandran C, Shenoi SD, Prabhu S. Clotheson PUVA in psoriasis: Single blind randomized comparative trial on 21 patients. Ind J Dermatol Venereol Leprol 2004;70:152–55.

9. Tiwari A, Srinivas CR, Musthafa M, Rai R, Surendran P. Installation of solarium-2000 for phototherapy. Ind J Dermatol Venereol Leprol 2003; 69:10–11.

10. Berneburg M, Herzinger T, Rampf J, et al. Efficacy of bath psoralen plus ultraviolet A (PUVA) vs. system PUVA in psoriasis: a prospective, open randomized multicentric study. Br J Dermatol 2013;169:704–8.

11. Luffle M, Degitz K, Plewig G, Rocken M. Psoralen bath plus UVA therapy possibilities and limitations. Arch Dermatol 1997;133:1597–603.

12. Calzavara-Pinton P, Ortel B, Carlino A, Honigsmann H, De Panfilis G. Phototesting and phototoxic side effects in bath PUVA. J Am Acad Dermatol 1993;28:657–9.

13. Fisher T, Alsins J. Treatment of psoriasis with trioxsalen baths and dysprosium lamps. Acta Derm Venereol 1976;56:383–90.

14. Sridhar KS, Srinivas CR, Shenoi SD. PUVA therapy for psoriasis, comparision of oral and bath water delivery of 8-MOP. Ind J Dermatol Venereol Leprol 1992;58:252–4.

15. Pai S, Srinivas CR. Bathing suit delivery of 8-methoxypsoralen in psoriasis: A double blind placebo controlled study. Int J Dermatol 1994; 33:576–8.

16. Van Weelden H, De La Faille HB, Young E, van der Leun JC. A new development in UVB phototherapy of psoriasis. Br J Dermatol 1988; 119:11–9.

17. Green C, Ferguson J, Lakshmipathi T, Johnson BE. 311 nm UVB phototherapy—an effective treatment for psoriasis. Br J Dermatol 1988;119:691–6.

18. Ibbotson SH, Bisland D, Cox NH, Dawe RS, et al. An update and guidance on narrowband ultraviolet B phototheapry: A British Photodermatology Group Workshop. Br J Dermatol 2004; 151:283–297.

19. Honigsmann H. UVB therapy (broadband and narrowband). In: UpToDate, Post TW (Ed), UpToDate, Elmets CA. (Accessed on August 15, 2015.)

20. Reich A, Medrek K. Effects of narrowband UVB (311) irradiation on epidermal cells. Int J Mol Sci 2013;14:8456–66.

21. Serish, Srinivas CR. Minimal erythema dose (Med) to narrow band ultraviolet-B (NB-UVB) broadband ultraviolet-B (BB-UVB): A pilot study. Indian J Dermatol Venereol Leprol 2002;68:63–64.

22. Pai GS, Vinod V, Krishna V. Med estimation for narrowband UV-B on type IV and type V skin in India. Indian J Dermatol Venereol Leprol 2002;68:140–41.
23. Tejasvi T, Sharma VK, Kaur J. Determination of minimal erythemal dose for narrowband-ultraviolet B radiation in north Indian patients: Comparison of visual and Dermaspectrometer® readings. Indian J Dermatol Venereol Leprol 2007;73:97–9.
24. Dawe RS, Cameron HM, Yule S, et al. A randomized comparison of methods of selecting NBUVB starting dose to treat chronic psoriasis. Arch Dermatol 2011;147:168–74.
25. Dogra S, De D. Narrowband ultraviolet B in the treatment of psoriasis: The journey so far! Indian J Dermatol Venereol Leprol 2010;76: 652–61.
26. Benakova N. Phototherapy for psoriasis. Acta Dermatovenerol Croat 2011;19(3):195–205.
27. Archier E, Devaux S, Castela E, Gallini A, et al. Efficacy of psoralen UVA therapy vs narrowband UVB therapy in chronic plaque psoriasis: a systematic literature review. J Eur Acad Dermatol Venereol 2012;26: 11–21.

15

Risk of Tuberculosis with TNF-α Antagonists

Kiran V Godse, Aayushi Mehta

TNF-α is a pro-inflammatory cytokine that plays an important role in the pathogenesis of psoriasis. Evidence has shown elevated levels of TNF-α in lesional skin as well as blood stream of psoriasis patients.[1]

Currently, three anti-TNF-α agents are FDA approved for use in psoriasis—infliximab, etanercept, adalimumab. Newer agents are golimumab and certolizumab, however, these are not yet FDA approved. All these agents are associated with an increased risk of reactivation of latent tuberculosis; this remains a major concern limiting their use in countries such as India where tuberculosis is a major problem.

ROLE OF TNF-α IN PROTECTION AGAINST TUBERCULOSIS[2-4]

TNF-α contributes to the control of tuberculosis by numerous mechanisms. The human host immune response to tuberculosis infection consists of macrophage activation and phagocytosis, activation of cell-mediated immunity, killing of mycobacteria and eventual granuloma formation to control the infection.

Granulomas are a hallmark of tuberculosis. These are immune microenvironments which contain the TB bacilli and prevent dissemination of infection. In many cases, these granulomas are also the sites for survival of bacilli for years inside these micro-environments, until conditions in the host favor reactivation. This is the so-called Latent Tuberculosis Infection (LTBI).

TNF-α in conjunction with IFN-γ activates macrophages which then phagocytose the bacilli. TNF is also critical in granuloma formation and maintenance. It mediates apoptosis of TB infected cells and recruits other cells for the immune response. Mouse models have shown that TNF-α has an important role to play in defence against TB bacilli, as described above.[5]

Incidence of TB Infection and Reactivation with Use of Biologics

TB is becoming an increasing problem, especially with the advent of HIV. It remains an endemic disease in India. As per the latest WHO data, the prevalence of TB, including HIV-TB coinfection, in India during the year 2013 was 211 per 1,00,000 population, making India a high TB burden nation.[6] A total of 12, 43, 905 new cases of TB were notified from India during the year 2013.[6]

The link between anti-TNF-α agents and TB had not been established until 2001,[7,8] when the first report was published, although infliximab was FDA approved since 1998 and many patients had already received the drug. Keane et al,[7] in their study, published data obtained by analysis of the FDA's adverse events reporting system. They showed that the reported frequency of tuberculosis in association with infliximab therapy was much higher than the frequency of other opportunistic infections.

Following this initial report, many studies were published recording the incidence of TB in patients receiving anti-TNF-α agents.[9–11]

In a study published in Indian population,[11] in 53 patients of inflammatory rheumatic diseases, 32% of the patients had one or more of the screening tests positive, with 5 of them having active TB infection (9.4%), and the remaining 22.6% being diagnosed as LTBI. Thus, this report reflects the much higher endemicity of TB in an Indian population compared to the other studies published in literature.[11]

As per a recently published Cochrane review[12] on the adverse effects of biologics, the odds ratio for tuberculosis reactivation with adalimumab was 2.14, with etanercept was 1.48, and with infliximab was 2.82. However, the authors felt that the quality of evidence in literature for the same was low.[12]

Differences in Risk Factors with Individual Anti-TNF-α Agents

Published literature and trials have consistently shown that there is a lower risk for TB with etanercept as compared to the other monoclonal antibodies (infliximab, adalimumab).[12,13] Data available for certolizumab and golimumab is limited.[13]

Evaluation of Patients who have Risk Factors for Tuberculosis

Risk factors for tuberculosis

History of tuberculosis in past

H/o recent exposure or contact to TB

Occupational exposure (healthcare workers)

Co-administration or past administration of other immunosuppressants

History of chronic cough, chest pains, weight loss, evening fever

HIV positivity

RECOMMENDATIONS FOR SCREENING OF LTBI

All patients who have immune-mediated inflammatory diseases, including dermatologic conditions such as psoriasis, and are candidates for anti-TNF-α therapy, should be screened for tuberculosis. This has been recommended by all currently available international guidelines.[13–15]

It has also been recommended that ideally the screening should be done at the initial diagnosis of the disease, because of some of the diseases themselves (such as rheumatoid arthritis and psoriasis) as well as chronic immunosuppressive therapy with other agents (such as corticosteroids) can independently increase the risk of TB.[15] In addition, therapy with chronic immunosuppressive agents may modify the results of the tuberculin skin test,[15] as well as the interferon gamma release assays (IGRAs).[16]

There is currently no available single confirmatory diagnostic test for LTBI. There are various recommendations and guidelines published in literature about screening and management; however, there remains a paucity of studies from India which is a high TB burden nation.

It is generally agreed upon that the combination of both a TST and an IGRA offer the best chance for highest sensitivity and specificity of detecting LTBI.

So far, there has been only one publication in an Indian population, evaluating strategies for preventing tuberculosis flares in patients who may receive treatment with TNF-α inhibitors.[11] The screening protocol followed by them included use of an initial TST, IGRA, as well as chest X-ray, and additional use of a CT chest in all cases where chest X-ray findings were equivocal. Using these 4 tests for screening, the authors hoped to minimize the incidence of TB. Out of the 53 patients screened, 22 went on to receive anti-TNF-α treatment, and 1 of them, in spite of being negative in all the screening tests, eventually developed tuberculosis.[11] However, by using this screening protocol, the percentage of patients developing tuberculosis went down from 18% to 4.5%.

Currently available WHO guidelines for screening and management of LTBI, recommend that all individuals should first be asked about symptoms of active TB and active foci should be ruled out by CXR and other investigations as necessary. Following this, although WHO recommends use of either TST or an IGRA for screening of TB, most published literature and clinical experience, especially from India, would suggest that sensitivity and specifity is improved by a combination of both these tests.[11,14,15]

INTERPRETING THE TUBERCULIN SKIN TEST (TST)

Malaviya et al,[11] in their study, used 10 TU for the TST, in order to compensate for the immunocompromised status of most study subjects. However, most guidelines for TST testing recommend use of 5 TU of PPD. The results can be interpreted as:

≥ 5 mm for persons at high risk of developing TB (HIV, immuno-suppression, close contact with infected person)

≥ 10 mm for persons with increased probability of recent infection or other risk factors (e.g. high-prevalence TB countries, diabetes mellitus)

≥ 15 mm in persons at low risk for TB.

Routinely ≥ 10 mm is the cut-off used in India for most of the population. The routine BCG vaccination everyone receives has been said to lead to a higher rate of false positives with TST, emphasising the need for combining with other screening tools including IGRAs, chest X-ray and clinical history.

MANAGEMENT OF LTBI AND ACTIVE INFECTIONS

All active cases of TB require to complete the 6 months course of treatment with WHO-MDT for TB, and biologic therapy is not initiated during this period.

Once detected, LTBI in patients who are candidates for anti-TNF-α therapy must be treated and prophylaxis initiated before starting the biologic. The WHO recommends treatment of LTBI in the form of 6 or 9 months of isoniazid alone, or 3 to 4 months of isoniazid plus rifampicin.

Most studies published from Western countries have recommended treatment with isoniazid for 4 months before starting anti-TNF treatment. However, in the Indian study conducted by Malaviya et al,[11] the patients who were detected with LTBI received treatment in the form of both isoniazid plus rifampicin. TNF-α antagonists were initiated after 2 months of prophylaxis. Those patients with active TB (after completion of MDT) as well as those with LTBI were continued on isoniazid plus rifampicin throughout the duration of treatment with TNF-antagonist, and up to 2 months after stopping of treatment.[11] The authors recommended use of the two-drug regimen to prevent development of resistance and improve efficacy.

While many authors recommend completing the entire duration of the prophylaxis before initiating anti-TNF therapies, others recommend initiation of anti-TNF therapy after 1–2 months of prophylaxis if the clinical condition so warrants.[17]

Conclusion

Screening for latent tuberculosis infection is mandatory in all patients who might receive anti-TNF therapies. Ideally the screening should be done at diagnosis itself. Screening may consist of only TST or a combination of TST with IGRA depending on availability of these tests, in combination with clinical history, evaluation, and chest X-ray. In cases with doubtful findings on chest X-ray, a CT chest may be used to distinguish active TB. All cases of LTBI should receive treatment for minimum 1 to 2 months before initiating anti-TNF therapy, and throughout the duration of treatment.

REFERENCES

1. Yost J, Gudjonsson JE. The role of TNF inhibitors in psoriasis therapy: new implications for associated comorbidities. F1000 Medicine Reports 2009;1:30 (doi: 10.3410/M1-30).

2. Lin PL, Plessner HL, Voitenok NN, Flynn JL. Tumor Necrosis Factor and Tuberculosis. Journal of Investigative Dermatology Symposium Proceedings 2007;12:22–5.

3. Stenger S. Immunological control of tuberculosis: role of tumour necrosis factor and more. Ann Rheum Dis 2005;64(4):iv24–8.

4. Bhargava K. Anti-TNF-alpha Therapy and Tuberculosis: Theoretical and Practical Considerations. International Journal of Clinical Reviews 2010, p.12.

5. Flynn JL, et al. Tumor necrosis factor-alpha is required in the protective immune response against *Mycobacterium tuberculosis* in mice. Immunity 1995;2:561–72.

6. WHO TB Data: Tuberculosis country profiles (Epidemiology and Strategy). Accessed from: *https://extranet.who.int/sree/Reports%?op=Replet and name=%2FWHO_HQ_Reports%2FG2% 2FPROD%2FEXT%2FTB CountryProfile and ISO2=IN and LAN=EN and outtype=html.* Last accessed: 30 September 2015.

7. Keane J, Gershon S, Robert PW, Mirabile-Levens E, Kasznica J, Schwieterman WD, et al. Tuberculosis associated with infliximab, a tumor necrosis factor (alpha)-neutralizing agent. N Engl J Med 2001; 345(15):1098–104.

8. Sivamani RK, Goodarzi H, Garcia MS, Raychaudhuri SP, Wehrli LN, Ono Y, et al. Biologic Therapies in the Treatment of Psoriasis: A Comprehensive Evidence-Based Basic Science and Clinical Review and a Practical Guide to Tuberculosis Monitoring. Clin Rev Allergy Immunol 2013;44(2):121–40.

9. Mankia S, Peters JE, Kang S, Moore S, Ehrenstein MR. Tuberculosis and anti-TNF treatment: experience of a central London hospital. Clin Rheumatol 2011;30(3):399–401.

10. Medina-Gil C, Dehesa L, Vega A, Kerdel F. Prevalence of latent tuberculosis infection in patients with moderate to severe psoriasis taking biologic therapies in a dermatologic private practice in Miami, Florida. Int J Dermatol 2015;54(7):846–52.

11. Malaviya AN, Kapoor S, Garg S, Rawat R, Shankar S, Nagpal S, et al. Preventing tuberculosis flare in patients with inflammatory rheumatic diseases receiving tumor necrosis factor-alpha inhibitors in India—An audit report. J Rheumatol 2009;36(7):1414–20.

12. Singh JA, Wells GA, Christensen R, Maxwell LJ, Skoetz N, Tugwell P, et al. Adverse effects of biologics: a network meta-analysis and Cochrane overview. Cochrane Database of Systematic Reviews 2011; Issue 2. Art. No. CD008794.

13. Cantini F, Nannini C, Niccoli L, Iannone F, Delogu G, Garlaschi G. SAFEBIO (Italian multidisciplinary task force for screening of tuberculosis before and during biologic therapy). Guidance for the management of patients with latent tuberculosis infection requiring biologic therapy in rheumatology and dermatology clinical practice. Autoimmun Rev 2015;14(6):503–9.

14. Hewitt RJ, Francis M, Singanayagam A, Kon OM. Screening tests for tuberculosis before starting biological therapy. BMJ 2015;350:h1060.

15. Duarte R, Campainha S, Cotter J, Rosa B, Varela P, Correia A, et al. Position paper on tuberculosis screening in patients with immune mediated inflammatory diseases candidates for biological therapy. Acta Reumatol Port 2012;37(3):253–9.

16. Clifford V, Tebruegge M, Curtis N. Limitations of current tuberculosis screening tests in immunosuppressed patients. BMJ 2015 Apr 28; 350:h2226.

17. Gardam MA, Keystone EC, Menzies R, Manners S, Skamene E, et al. Anti-tumour necrosis factor agents and tuberculosis risk: mechanisms of action and clinical management. Lancet Infect Dis 2003;3(3): 148–55.

16

Biologics in Psoriasis

Vidya Kharkar

Biologics, also known as biologic therapies or biological response modifiers, are drugs derived from living material (human, plant, animal, or micro-organism). They interfere with specific parts of the body's immune system to treat and prevent immune-mediated inflammatory disorders and cancers. They are also called targeted therapies.

How do biologics work in psoriasis?
- Evidence strongly suggests that psoriasis is a disorder of the immune system.
- Abnormally large numbers of T-cells trigger the release of cytokines that can cause inflammation, redness, itching and flaky skin patches characteristic of psoriasis.
- Biologics work by interfering with specific components of the autoimmune response.

Advantages over general immunosuppressants
- General immunosuppressants, suppress the entire immune system
- Biologics can fight more selectively and target only those chemicals involved in causing psoriasis

Biologics

Type	Drugs
T-cell activation inhibitors	Alefacept, efalizumab, abatacept
TNF-α antagonists	Infliximab, adalimumab, etanercept, golimumab, certolizumab

| Anti IL 12/23 antibodies | Ustekinumab, briakinumab |
| IL-17/IL-17R inhibitors | Secukinumab, ixekizumab, Brodalumab |

Which patients should be considered eligible for treatment?

- Most patients with moderate to severe disease achieve satisfactory disease control in the short term with at least one of the systemic agents.
- Long-term disease control frequently requires some form of continuous therapy and consequent, predictable risks of toxicity.
- At present, the risks and benefits of biologic therapies relative to standard systemic therapy are largely unknown.
- Widespread use of these agents in uncomplicated moderate to severe psoriasis is inappropriate and is not supported by the licensed indications for these drugs.

When should biologics be used?

Due to the high cost of these medicines, their use is limited to patients with moderate to severe psoriasis where:

- All other treatments have failed
- Side effects of other treatments become intolerable or toxicity has occurred
- Concurrent diseases such as congestive heart failure or liver disease and associated comorbidites

RECOMMENDATIONS

Eligibility criteria: To be considered eligible for treatment. Patients must have severe disease as defined in (a) and fulfil one of the clinical categories outlined in (b):

(a) Severe disease defined as a PASI score of 10 or more (or a BSA of 10% or greater where PASI is not applicable) and a DLQI > 10.

- In exceptional circumstances (e.g. disease affecting high-impact sites with associated significant functional or psychological morbidity such as acral psoriasis, hands, feet, head, neck, genitalia with associated significant functional or psychological morbidity). AND

(b) Fulfil at least one of the following clinical categories

- Where phototherapy and alternative standard systemic therapy are contraindicated or cannot be used due to the development of, or risk of developing, clinically important treatment related toxicity.

- are intolerant to standard systemic therapy
- are unresponsive to standard systemic therapy

Use of biologic therapy in combination with phototherapy

- The rationale for using these two contrasting forms of treatment together is that both have different mechanisms of action which may be synergistic when used together.
- However, trial data are limited to a single arm, open-label study, evaluating etanercept 50 mg twice weekly combined with narrowband UVB phototherapy given three times weekly ($n = 86$).
- At week 12, 26% of patients achieved PASI 100, 58.1% achieved PASI 90, and 84.9% achieved PASI 75.
- It is unclear what effect each treatment had as this study failed to include a comparator group with either monotherapy or placebo.
- There is currently insufficient evidence to recommend the combination of narrowband UVB phototherapy with etanercept, and
- No data at all on combined use of infliximab or adalimumab with phototherapy.

Etanercept with MTX

Studies of Enbrel (etanercept) with methotrexate have shown a much improved response compared to etanercept alone.

Biologics and acitretin

Topical therapy and oral retinoids like acitretin may be used in combination with biologics for improved results.

How to determine the optimal choice and sequence of therapy

- TNF antagonists are recommended as first-line intervention for patients fulfilling criteria for treatment with biologic therapy
- The choice of which of the three TNF antagonists to used first should be based on clinical need and requires a careful assessment of risks and benefits of each agent in the context of the individual patient. With this provision, the following additional recommendations are made.

For patients with stable chronic plaque psoriasis

- Etanercept or adalimumab may be considered first choice based on the favorable risk–benefit profile and ease of administration.

For patients requiring rapid disease control
- Adalimumab or infliximab may be considered first choice due to the early onset of action, and high chance of achieving PASI 75 by 3 months.
- For patients with unstable or generalized pustular psoriasis.
  Limited evidence indicates that infliximab is effective and may therefore be considered as first choice.
- For patients who do not respond to a TNF antagonist (either primary or secondary failure), a second TNF antagonist may be considered.
- Due to the lack of patient-years exposure and long-term safety data limited to 1 year, ustekinumab should be reserved for use as a second-line biologic agent where TNF therapy has failed or cannot be used.

PRESCREENING FOR BIOLOGICS

Eligibility Criteria

I. Disease severity: PASI >/= 10
                      DLQI >/= 10
- Etanercept
- Adalimumab
- Ustekinumab

II. Disease severity: PASI >/= 20
                       DLQI >/= 18
- Infliximab

Previous systemic therapies:
- Methotrexate
- Cyclosporine
- Acitretin
- UVB
- PUVA

Reason for discontinuation, intolerance, toxicity, contra-indication and lack of efficacy.

Exclusion criteria

Absolute exclusion from therapy:
- Pregnancy/breastfeeding
- Active infection
- High risk of infection

- Multiple sclerosis
- Malignancy (excluding NMSC)

Requiring further discussion:
- Previous tuberculosis
- Congestive heart failure
- Diabetes mellitus
- PUVA >200 especially after cyclosporin
- HIV positive
- Hepatitis B or C

Physical Examination

- Check for demyelination, lymphadenopathy, hepato-splenomegaly.
- Skin check.

Investigations

- Chest X-ray
- Urine dip
- Blood: Complete blood count, urea and electrolytes, liver function tests, fasting lipids, anti-nuclear antibodies, HIV, varicella serology, hepatitis B and C, interferon gamma release assay (quantiferon gold/T-spot)

What are the indications for stopping therapy?
- Therapy should be discontinued when patients fail to achieve an adequate response following treatment initiation or when treatment response is not maintained.
- Withdrawal of therapy is also indicated due to the following events:
  - a serious adverse event. Serious adverse events which may justify the withdrawal of treatment include malignancy (excluding NMSC), severe drug-related toxicity, severe intercurrent infection (temporary withdrawal)
  - pregnancy (temporary withdrawal)
  - elective surgical procedures

What is the definition of a disease response?
- An adequate response to treatment is defined as either
  - a 50% or greater reduction in baseline PASI (PASI 50 response) and a 5-point or greater improvement in DLQI4, or

+ a 75% reduction in PASI score compared with baseline (PASI 75 response).

"Inadequate response": Is defined as:
- For whole body severe chronic plaque psoriasis
- a PASI score of greater than 15
- as assessed preferably while still on treatment but no longer than 1 month following cessation of the most recent prior treatment
- For severe chronic plaque psoriasis of the face, hand or foot,
- at least 2 of the 3 PASI symptom subscores for erythema, thickness and scaling are rated as severe or very severe, and
- The skin affected is 30% or more of the face, palm of a hand or sole of a foot, as assessed preferably while still on treatment but no longer than 1 month following cessation of the most recent prior treatment.

RECOMMENDED READING

1. Fernanda Bellodi Schmidt, Kara N Shah. Biologic Response Modifiers and Pediatric Psoriasis. Pediatric Dermatology 2015;32(3):33–320.
2. Jennifer C Cather, Jeffrey J Crowley. Use of Biologic Agents in Combination with Other Therapies for the Treatment of Psoriasis. Am J Clin Dermatol 2014;15:467–78.
3. Sehgal VN, Pandhi D, Khurana A. Biologics in dermatology: An integrated review. Indian J Dermatol 2014;59:425–41.

17

Dermoscopy in Psoriasis

Aditya Mahajan

INTRODUCTION

Psoriasis is a common inflammatory, chronic-relapsing, erythematous-desquamative dermatosis, which affects about 3% of the overall population of the world. The most common presentation is the chronic plaque type which consists of erythematous plaques with silvery white scales located over the extensor aspects of limbs, sacral area, scalp, palms and soles.

A dermoscope (dermatoscope) is a non-invasive, diagnostic tool which visualizes subtle clinical patterns of skin lesions and subsurface skin structures not normally visible to the unaided eye.[1]

Dermoscopy is known to be useful in evaluating skin tumors, but its applicability extends also to the field of inflammatory skin disorders like plaque psoriasis.

Though clinical diagnosis is mostly easy and straightforward in cases of psoriasis, sometimes it can be confusing and various differentials have to be considered. Dermoscopy can prove to be an efficient tool in such scenarios. Also it aides in therapeutic planning.

DERMOSCOPY IN PSORIASIS

Before going to the dermoscopy it is important to understand the histopathology of psoriatic plaque. Epidermis shows hyper-keratosis, microabscesses of Munro in the horny layer and spongiform pustules of Kagoj. There is elongation and camel footing of rete ridges. The papillary dermis shows dilated, twisted capillaries. It is this vascular pattern that is better visualized in the dermoscopy of psoriasis.

The dermoscopy (10x) of an established plaque of psoriasis shows dotted or pinpoint red capillaries appearing as red dots which represent the "top view" of the dermal dilated, twisted capillaries. Apart from this thick silvery white scaling is also visualized[2] (Figs 17.1 and 17.2). According to Francesco Lacarrubba et al. it is necessary to distinguish these red dots from other conditions in which red dots are seen like eczema, lichen planus, pityriasis rosea, pityriasis rubra pilaris, porokeratosis, in which the distribution of the red dots is not uniform over the area and there is presence of coexisting features like yellow scales in eczema, Wickham's striae in lichen planus, yellowish background color in pityriasis rosea, etc.

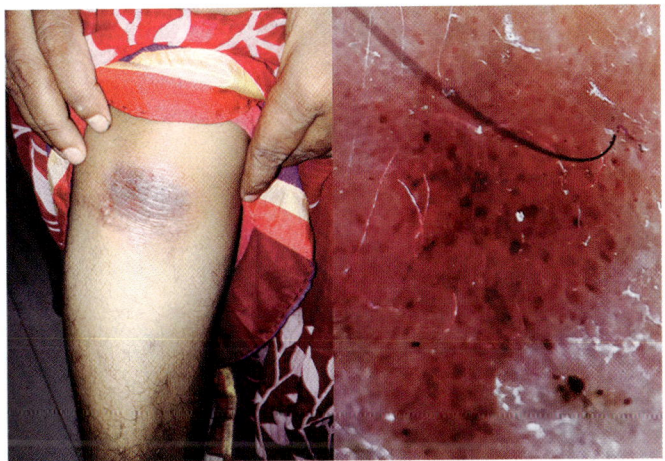

Fig. 17.1 Dermoscopy of a plaque of psoriasis (10x) showing multiple red dots

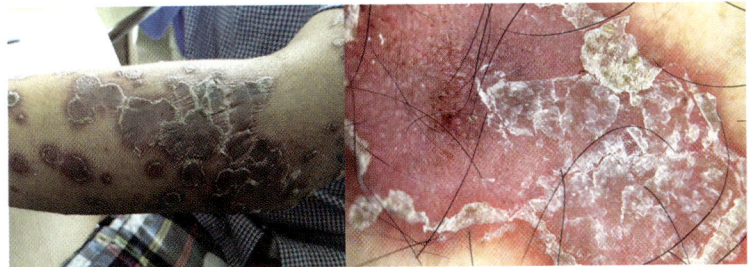

Fig. 17.2 A case of chronic plaque psoriasis showing silvery white scaling along with red dots on dermoscopy (10x)

On higher magnification (100x) the specific pattern of these dilated capillaries is visualized; which can be bushy, hairpin like (hairpin seen mainly over the edges of the lesion). Using video-dermoscopy the diameter of these capillaries can be calculated. It is 50–110 μm which is more than normal (Fig. 17.3).

Such patterns of red dots, globules and twisted capillaries are also observed on scalp lesions.

In palmoplantar lesions it can be difficult to observe changes due to extensive hyperkeratosis. But changes similar to chronic plaque psoriasis can be observed in areas with lesser scaling (Fig. 17.4).

Nail psoriasis shows a pinkish yellow border which surrounds the area of onycholysis along with splinter hemorrhages. Nail dermoscopy helps to distinguish nail psoriasis from onycho-mycosis (Fig. 17.5).

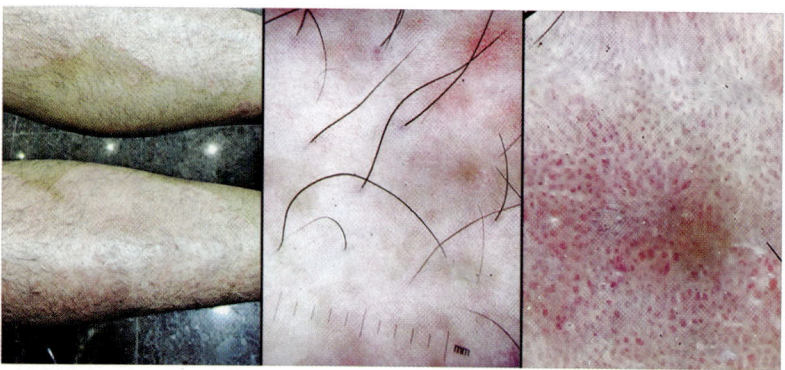

Fig. 17.3 Dermoscopy (10x and 100x) showing red dots and "bushy" pattern of arrangement of capillaries in a plaque of psoriasis

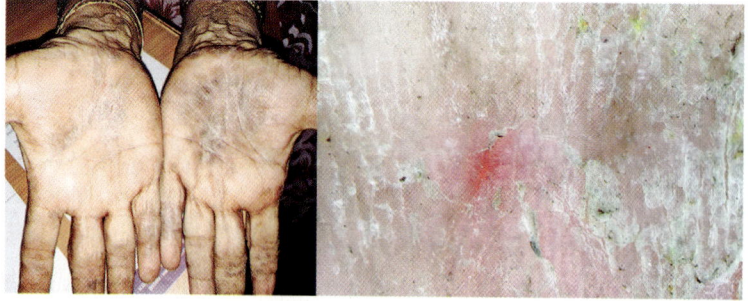

Fig. 17.4 Palmoplantar psoriasis

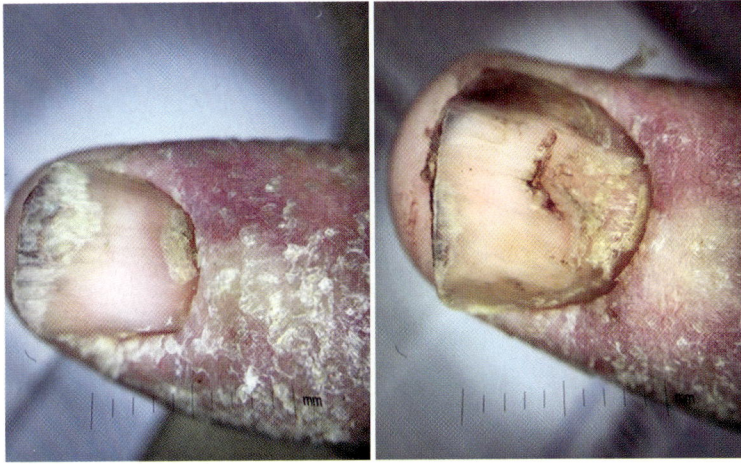

Fig. 17.5 Nail dermoscopy showing onycholysis surrounded by a pink yellow border. In the second photo splinter hemorrhages can be observed as three dots on the lower side of the nail plate

Pustular psoriasis shows multiple white pus containing vesicles, slight erythema. Vascular changes are not so prominent in pustular psoriasis; correlating to the histopathological findings (Figs 17.6 and 17.7).

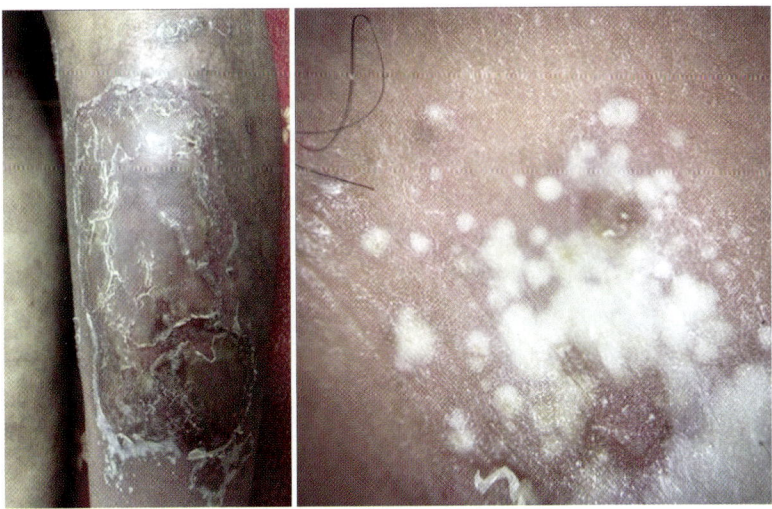

Fig. 17.6 A case of pustular psoriasis; dermoscopy (10x) shows multiple pus-filled lesions

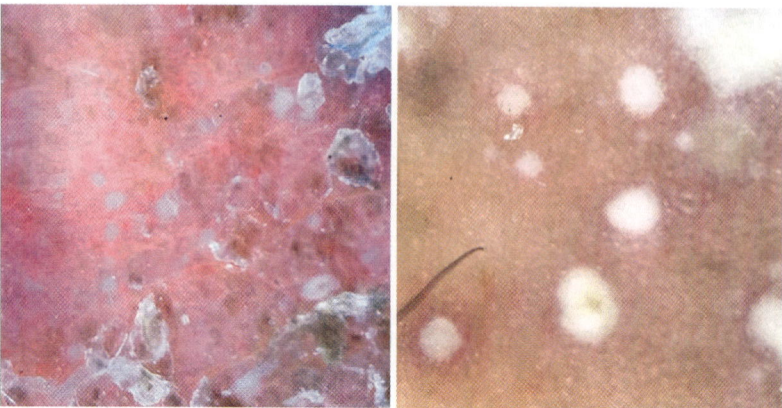

Fig. 17.7 On higher magnification slight erythema is seen along with pus-filled lesions of pustular psoriasis

DERMOSCOPY FOR EVALUATION OF TREATMENT

Dermoscopy also proves to be useful in assessing treatment, deciding on when to stop or taper therapy.[3] There is decrease in erythema along with decrease in dilation of the capillaries. None of the patients return to a completely normal dermoscopic pattern.[4] The cutaneous microcirculation continues to be affected in spite of clinical cure of disease.[5]

Conclusion

To conclude, dermoscope can be considered a useful and easy to use tool for the diagnosis of psoriasis. Its use in prognosis and treatment is also well established. Dermoscopy needs to be done when there is clearance of skin lesions and decision regarding cessation or tapering of therapy has to be considered.

REFERENCES

1. Nischal K C, Khopkar U. Dermoscope. Indian J Dermatol Venereol Leprol 2005; 71:300–3.
2. Lacarrubba F, Verzì AE and Micali G. Dermatoscopy and Video Dermatoscopy in the Diagnosis and Therapeutic Monitoring of Plaque Psoriasis: A Review. Austin J Dermatolog. 2014;1(6):1030.

3. Lacarrubba F, D'Amico V, Nasca MR, Dinotta F, Micali G. Use of dermatoscopy and video dermatoscopy in therapeutic follow-up: A review. Int J Dermatol 2010; 49:866–873.
4. Stinco G, Buligan C, Maione V, Valent F, Patrone P. Video capillaroscopic findings in the microcirculation of the psoriatic plaque during etanercept therapy. Clin Exp Dermatol 2013; 38:633–637.
5. Stinco G, Lautieri S, Valent F, Patrone P. Cutaneous vascular alterations in psoriatic patients treated with cyclosporine. Acta Derm Venereol 2007; 87:152–154.

18

Palmoplantar Psoriasis

Sujay Khandpur

Palmoplantar psoriasis (PPP) is the localized form of psoriasis. It accounts for 3–4% of all psoriasis cases and produces significant functional and social disability. In a recent study it was shown that the effect of palmoplantar psoriasis on the quality of patients is much worse than plaque psoriasis.[1] It is a chronic recurring condition that may exist in the absence of typical psoriatic lesions elsewhere on the body.

EPIDEMIOLOGY

The prevalence of psoriasis of the palms and soles varies widely in different studies, ranging from 2.8% to 40.9% of psoriasis cases.[2–4] In a study from Chandigarh, India, of 3065 patients of psoriasis having been screened; palmar or plantar lesions were present in 540 (17.6%) patients.[2] In a study from South India in which 403 psoriasis patients were studied, palmoplantar involvement was seen in 59% cases.[3] In a recent classification of psoriasis proposed by Guinot et al., type 2 phenotype is characterized by palmoplantar involvement and constitutes about 7% of the total patient population.[4]

The most common affected age group is 20–50 years of age.[2,5] Majority of the Indian studies have shown a male predominance, although a few have shown equal sex predilection.[2,3,5] The most common occupation of affected individuals has been observed to be manual laborers, followed by housewives and farmers.[2,3,5] Pressure sites are commonly affected in these patients. This suggests the role of Koebner's phenomenon in the causation of palmoplantar psoriasis.

CLINICAL FEATURES

Hyperkeratotic, erythematous, scaly, fissured plaques are the commonest presentation. Pustular lesions are seen in palmoplantar pustulosis which is not considered as a subtype of palmoplantar psoriasis in the recent classification.

Site of Involvement

Of 154 cases with palmoplantar involvement in psoriasis, we had noticed involvement of both palms and soles in majority of the patients (48%), with 15% each having involvement of either palms or soles.[5] Kumar et al. had observed both palmoplantar involvement in 47.5% of the patients, followed by plantar psoriasis in 44.3% and palmar psoriasis only in 8.1% patients.[2] This can probably be attributed to the Indian custom of walking barefoot.

The sites of involvement are typically over the pressure bearing areas such as center of the palm, thenar and hypothenar eminences, volar aspect of fingers, heels, instep and center of the sole. Localization of the lesions over pressure sites has been shown to be significantly associated with occupation and more common in manual laborers.[2] Extension of the lesion on to the dorsa of the hands and feet may occur in 43–68% of patients and is more common with palmar involvement than plantar.[2,5] Involvement of the interdigital areas is very variable and has been observed in 3.5% to 28% cases in different studies.[2,5] Involvement of the interdigital spaces of the feet is termed 'psoriasis alba'. In a cross-sectional analysis of 232 psoriatic patients, 22 (9.5%) patients had palmoplantar involvement and 2.6% of these showed involvement of interdigital spaces.[6] Linear crateriform lesions along the margins of the hands have also been reported.[7]

Well defined, discrete plaques are the most common morphological feature, although diffuse keratoderma may occur in 22–32% of palmoplantar psoriasis cases.[2] This has also shown a significant association with the type of work, as diffuse keratoderma was recorded predominantly in manual laborers. This observation supports the role of pressure in the causation and aggravation of palmoplantar psoriasis.

Symmetry of the Lesions

The lesions of PPP are typically bilaterally symmetrical, although unilateral involvement may be seen on the dominant hand of manual workers. In our study, the lesions were symmetrically distributed in 79% of cases.[5] Kumar et al. noticed unilateral involvement of the palm in 3.8% patients and the sole in 3.7% patients.[2] Palmar involvement had a right-hand predominance and was mostly seen in male manual laborers, but unilateral plantar involvement was not specifically associated with any site, gender or occupation.[2,5]

Associated Psoriatic Plaques at Other Sites

Palmoplantar psoriasis can occur in the absence of psoriatic plaques elsewhere on the body in 21–70% of cases, which may reflect a high incidence of "pure" palmoplantar disease, or the longer persistence/refractory nature of lesions at these sites.[2–5] Kumar et al. noticed typical psoriatic lesions elsewhere on the body in only 30.3% of the patients; 94% of these had plaque-type psoriasis and 4% had scalp lesions.[2]

Associated Nail Involvement

Nail findings in psoriasis include nail matrix signs such as pitting, leuconychia, red lunula and crumbling of the nail plate and nail bed findings such as onycholysis, splinter hemorrhages, oil-drop sign and subungual hyperkeratosis. We reviewed 154 patients of palmoplantar psoriasis and found associated nail involvement in 41% cases.[5] Most common findings were coarse pitting (30 patients), subungual hyperkeratosis (24 cases), and longitudinal ridging (18 patients). Chopra et al. reviewed 64 cases of palmoplantar psoriasis and reported nail involvement in 23.4% of cases.[8]

Associated Joint Involvement

A peripheral monoarticular or asymmetric oligoarticular arthritis is the commonest form of joint involvement in psoriasis. We observed joint pain and swelling, suggestive of arthritis, in nine of 154 (5.8%) palmoplantar psoriasis cases.[5] Ferrandiz et al. noticed joint involvement in 17% of their palmoplantar psoriasis cases.[9] Psoriatic arthritis was diagnosed in 9.4% cases and joint deformity was present in 5% patients.

SYMPTOMS

Palmoplantar psoriasis is usually symptomatic (73.7–81.8%).[2,3] The commonest symptoms include pain, itching, irritation and fissuring. Plantar lesions may result in discomfort during walking and fissuring may result in secondary infection. Palmar lesions make household works difficult. In view of the involvement of exposed sites, a high psychosocial burden is noticed.[10]

Seasonal Variation

Winter exacerbation is seen in majority of the cases, with reduced severity in summer.[2]

Severity Score

Brunasso et al. proposed a modified palmoplantar pustular psoriasis area and severity index (m-PPPASI), which has been found to be a useful scoring system in the monitoring of treatment response in palmoplantar psoriasis.[10] The m-PPPASI score evaluates the area of psoriatic involvement and the severity for each of the three clinical skin signs: erythema, infiltration (for plaque PPP) or pustules (for pustular PPP) and desquamation (Table 18.1).

Diagnosis of Palmoplantar Psoriasis

The diagnosis of this condition usually depends on the characteristics morphology and location of the lesions. Histopathology may show overlapping features with other disorders. The most

Table 18.1: m-PPPASI scoring system

Skin sign	Right palm	Left palm	Right sole	Left sole
Erythema	Score from 0 to 4	Score from 0 to 4	Score from 0 to 4	Score from 0 to 4
Infiltration	Score from 0 to 4	Score from 0 to 4	Score from 0 to 4	Score from 0 to 4
Desquamation	Score from 0 to 4	Score from 0 to 4	Score from 0 to 4	Score from 0 to 4
Total clinical severity	Max:12	Max:12	Max:12	Max:12
Extent of involvement	0 = none, $1 \leq 10\%$, 2 = 10 to <30%, 3 = 30 to <50%, 4 = 50 to <70%, 5 = 70–90% and 6 = 90–100%			
Total extent of involvement	Max = 6 × 0.20	Max = 6 × 0.20	Max = 6 × 0.30	Max = 6 × 0.30
Multiply total extent of involvement and total clinical severity	A (Max = 14.4)	B (Max = 14.4)	C (Max = 21.6)	D (Max = 21.6)
Total m-PPPASI	A + B + C + D, max = 72			

important differential diagnosis clinically and histologically is hyperkerartotic dermatitis of the palms and soles.

Clinically, well-defined, symmetrically distributed, hyperkeratotic, dry, fissured plaques, involvement of the pressure-bearing sites including knuckles and interphalangeal joints are important clues to the diagnosis of palmoplantar psoriasis. Eczematous lesions are usually ill-defined and asymmetrical in distribution without predilection for pressure sites and sometimes associated with historical or clinical evidence of exudation during the course of the disease. The presence of psoriasis elsewhere or typical nail changes further support the diagnosis of palmoplantar psoriasis.

Other clinical differential diagnoses include pityriasis rubra pilaris (PRP), Reiter's disease, erythrokeratodermia, allergic contact dermatitis, tinea manuum, tinea pedis (moccasin-foot variant) and lichen planus. Pityriasis rubra pilaris results in a diffuse, waxy, yellow-orange keratoderma of the palms and soles. Cephalocaudal progression of skin lesions, presence of follicular papules and skip areas point towards the diagnosis.

Reiter's disease or reactive arthritis is characterized by keratoderma blennorrhagicum, which is seen more on the soles than palms. It starts as a dull red macule which rapidly becomes papular and pseudovesicular. Its color changes from yellow to orange-red as the roof thickens to form a hyperkaratotic plaque. Associated findings include urethritis, arthritis and conjunctivitis, rupioid hyperkeratotic skin lesions, nail dystrophy usually without nail pitting and circinate balanitis. Progressive symmetric erythrokeratodermia, an autosomal dominant inherited disorder, is characterised by yellowish thickening and desquamation of the palms and soles. It is also associated with symmetrically distributed, fixed or slowly progressive erythematous, scaly plaques over the shoulder girdle, cheeks, buttocks, knees and elbows. Unilateral involvement is a clue towards the diagnosis of tinea manuum and pedis. Lichen planus on the palms and soles presents as discrete, yellowish, punctuate to larger papules and plaques, sometimes wih overlying pits, though presence of violaceous papular lesions elsewhere, characteristic involvement of nails, scalp and mucosa may help in the diagnosis.

Histology may help to differentiate these conditions from palmoplantar psoriasis. Histological findings are usually identical in both psoriasis and hyperkeratotic eczema, but there are a few subtle differentiating points. Spongiosis, a characteristic feature of eczema, has been seen in palmoplantar psoriasis patients.[11] In a cross-sectional study of 52 patients (palmoplantar psoriasis: n=36, palmoplantar eczema: n=16), hypogranulosis, Munro's micro-abscess, tortuous blood vessels in papillary dermis, thinning of suprapapillary plate, confluent parakeratosis and spongiform pustule of Kogoj were the significant findings in psoriasis. Plasma mounds were significantly associated with palmoplantar eczema.[12] In another study, regular epidermal hyperplasia and marked parakeratosis were more frequent in palmoplantar psoriasis than in dermatitis. A study suggested presence of irregular epidermal hyperplasia and the detection of a higher number of S100-positive dendritic cells being in favor of dermatitis over psoriasis.[13] Aydin et al. analyzed 17 patients of palmoplantar psoriasis and 25 of eczematous dermatitis and noticed that confluent parakeratosis was more common in eczematous dermatitis while multiple foci of parakeratosis were common in psoriasis. Vertically situated multiple foci of parakeratosis, alternating with orthokeratosis, was the only statistically significant feature in favor of psoriasis. An interesting finding in this study was the presence of spongiotic vesicles in 76.5% of psoriasis patients. Presence of dyskeratotic cells was more common in psoriasis than in dermatitis, though not statistically significant.[11]

In a recent study, genetic analysis was performed in 28 eczema and 25 psoriasis cases. In general, they found that genes specific to psoriasis were important regulators of glucose and lipid metabolism while those specific to eczema were related to epidermal barrier and reduced innate immunity. From further analysis, they selected two genes—NOS2 and CCL27—that they considered would make a reliable classifier of disease.[14] NOS2 encodes for the inducible nitric oxidase synthase catalysing the production of nitric oxide (NO) and as such playing an important role in metabolic and inflammatory processes. It has been shown that disease activity of psoriasis correlates with dendritic cells expressing TNF-α and NOS2. CCL27, the cutaneous T-cell attracting chemokine, is constitutively expressed by epidermal keratinocytes. It binds to chemokine receptor 10 on skin-homing T cells and plays a crucial role in T cell-mediated inflammation. Serum levels of CCL27 were seen elevated in sera of both psoriasis and eczema patients, however, only in eczema, levels correlated with the clinical severity score.[15] Thus, NOS2 and CCL27 gene expression may help in differentiating palmoplantar psoriasis from hyperkeratotic eczema.

Carlen et al. compared epidermal HLA-C expression in normal epidermis, eczema and psoriasis cases and found that normal and eczematous tissue showed stronger expression of HLA-C than plaque psoriasis. Immunoreactivity in plaque psoriasis was consistently stronger in the basal layer, especially at the tips of rete ridges, while staining was seen in suprabasal keratinocytes of normal and eczema cases. This pattern may be explored further as a differentiating tool between these two conditions.[16]

In PRP, histological examination shows hyperkeratosis, alternating parakeratosis and orthokeratosis, acanthotic epidermis and prominent granular layer. Reiter's disease shows histological features identical to pustular psoriasis. Erythrokeratodermia shows hyperkeratosis, foci of parakeratosis, acanthotic epidermis with preserved granular layer. Lichen planus shows basal cell degeneration, necrotic keratinocytes, colloid bodies and lichenoid infiltrate in the papillary dermis.[17]

TREATMENT

The treatment modalities have to be titrated according to the disease severity and impact of the disease on daily activities. Topical, systemic or a combination of treatment scan be used.

Topical Therapy

Topical agents remain the most widely used treatment in palmoplantar psoriasis. These are of limited efficacy and best effective in the early or mild stage of the disease.

Topical steroids are the most commonly prescribed medications, and treatment under occlusion is known to improve the results. However, prolonged use of corticosteroids is associated with many adverse effects such as atrophy and depigmentation. In a retrospective analysis, superpotent steroid showed >50% reduction in disease in 31.6% of the patients.[11] Corticosteroids in conjunction with calcipotriol have shown greater efficacy than either therapies used alone and produce fewer side effects. It can be a treatment of choice for cases not responding to topical steroids alone. Use of calcipotriol under occlusion has also been shown to increase its efficacy in palmoplantar psoriasis.[18]

Coal tar has also been found useful in palmoplantar psoriasis. In a randomized controlled trial of 30 patients, 76.5% of patients showed significant improvement after 8 weeks of therapy.[19] Hence, combining topical steroid with coal tar may have an additive effect. Moreover, salicylic acid present in commercially available coal tar ointments improves the penetration of the medication, thereby enhancing the efficacy of the drug.[20]

Topical retinoids have also been used in combination with topical steroid to circumvent adverse effects and provide a synergistic effect. Tazarotene is the preferred topical retinoid in this condition. In a randomized controlled trial of 30 adult patients of palmoplantar psoriasis who were randomized to once daily application of topical tazarotene cream (0.1%) or once daily application of clobetasol propionate cream (0.05%) for 12 weeks, similar efficacy with significant improvement was seen in both the groups.[21] In the tazarotene treated group of 17 patients, 53% showed complete clearance (100% improvement), 17.6% showed excellent response (75–99% improvement), 23.5% showed good response (50–74% improvement) and 5.9% showed less than 50% improvement, while in the clobetasol treated group of 13 patients, 61.5% showed complete clearance (100% improvement), 15.4% showed excellent response (75–99% improvement) and 23% showed good response (50–74% improvement). In the tazarotene group, itching and irritation were complained by 6 (35.3%) and 4 patients (23.5%) at 2 and 4 weeks, respectively, which was self-limiting, while 53.8% of clobetasol treated patients developed hypopigmentation at the site of application.

Topical PUVA, administered as PUVA soaks or paint, has also shown good results. In a randomized controlled trial of 52 palmoplantar psoriasis cases, patients were randomized to receive either a combination of clobetasol propionate cream and coal tar daily (group 1) or topical PUVAsol on alternate days (group 2) for 16 weeks.[22] Both treatment groups had comparable efficacy at 16 weeks, with good improvement. Improvement in palmar lesions was observed in 90% cases in the topical steroid and coal tar group and in 75% cases in the topical PUVAsol group; for the soles, these figures were 76% and 79%, respectively. Kaur et al. evaluated the efficacy of topical PUVAsol in palmoplantar psoriasis and found 58.5% improvement in palmar and 43.5% reduction in plantar lesions after 8 weeks.[23]

PUVA soaks were used in 80 patients of palmoplantar psoriasis with a thrice weekly schedule and 56 patients completed at least 20 treatments.[24] Of these, 59% patients had an excellent response,

42% had minimal to moderate response and 29% had poor response. In resistant cases, the addition of acitretin to topical PUVA has shown significantly better response in a short time. In a study of 48 patients of palmoplantar psoriasis, 25 patients were treated with only topical PUVAsol and 17 patients with a combination regimen containing acitretin (10–25 mg/day).[25] Good response was seen in both the groups (65% in group 1 and 60% in group 2). It was concluded that adjunctive therapy with acitretin produces satisfactory results in a subset of patients in whom topical PUVA therapy alone would have failed. The main advantage of topical PUVA over oral PUVA is the avoidance of potential side effects of systemic therapy; therefore, topical PUVA is preferred in patients with hepatic or gastrointestinal diseases and cataract.

In a recent study, 10 patients with psoriasis of the palms and soles were randomly assigned to receive topical PUVA on one side and monochromatic excimer light 308 nm UVB on the contralateral side.[26] Both test groups showed remarkable PASI score reduction after 5 weeks. (308 nm UVB, 63.57%; cream PUVA, 64.64%). Monochromatic excimer light therapy was found to be an equally effective and convenient therapy for palmoplantar psoriasis.

Systemic Treatment

Chronic, severe, disabling and unresponsive disease may require systemic treatment. In a retrospective analysis, systemic treatment was required in 72.5% of palmoplantar cases.[18]

Retinoids are the most frequently used oral agents and are recommended as first-line systemic therapy, except in women of childbearing age. Acitretin is used in the dose of 25–50 mg per day. In a retrospective analysis of 114 patients of palmoplantar psoriasis, 53% patients had a 75% reduction in their disease from baseline after 8 weeks of treatment.[18] It can be administered alone or in combination with PUVA.

Oral PUVA alone or in combination with oral retinoids, can be used in resistant cases. Eight patients with moderate-to-severe psoriasis on sole and/or palms were randomly assigned to receive bath PUVA treatment on one side and oral PUVA on the other, three times a week for 4 weeks. After 4 weeks, both groups showed marked reduction in severity index (bath PUVA: 44%, oral PUVA: 52%).[27]

In view of thicker skin over palms and soles, PUVA is preferred over narrowband (NB-UVB) for palmoplantar psoriasis. In a study which included 25 cases, NB-UVB was compared with PUVA therapy, with local NB-UVB irradiation being given on one side and local PUVA on the other, three times a week for 9 weeks. The percentage reduction in the severity index score on PUVA-paint-treated side was 85.45% compared to 61.08% on the NB-UVB treated side, suggesting that PUVA therapy is superior to NBUVB therapy in this condition.[28]

Oral methotrexate has been used in doses of 20–30 mg per week in resistant cases of palmoplantar psoriasis. In a retrospective analysis of 114 patients, 47% cases showed significant improvement, i.e. > 75% reduction in their disease as compared to baseline after 4 months of methotrexate therapy.[18] Another retrospective analysis of 16 patients reported significant response in only one-third of patients receiving methotrexate, 15–25 mg per week, while 58% patients on acitretin, 10–25 mg daily, showed marked improvement (decrease in disease severity between 75 and 90%).[29] In a prospective randomized study, 111 patients of psoriasis with significant palmoplantar involvement were divided into two groups: Group I received methotrexate (0.4 mg D kg weekly) and Group II received acitretin (0.5 mg D kg daily). Marked improvement (m-PPPASI 75) was achieved in 24% patients in methotrexate group compared with 8% in acitretin group after 12 weeks, which was statistically significant (p = 0.029).[30]

In a study, 0.25% topical hydrogel form of methotrexate was found to be ineffective. It was attributed to the low absorption rates of the agent in the palmoplantar area.[31]

Low dose oral cyclosporine (2.5 mg/kg/day) for 12 weeks was used in 33 patients of palmoplantar psoriasis, which was increased to 5 mg/kg/day for next 12 weeks, 84% of patients showed significant improvement (defined as at least 50% reduction in disease severity) at the end of the therapeutic phase.[32]

The efficacy of colchicine in palmoplantar psoriasis is doubtful and it has been mainly used in palmoplantar pustulosis. Two randomized controlled trials showed conflicting results in palmoplantar pustulosis, though some studies have documented its efficacy.[33,34] In a retrospective analysis of 114 patients of palmoplantar psoriasis, 60% of colchicine (1–2 mg/day) users showed significant improvement with >75% reduction in disease after a mean of 4.5 ± 4 (1–12) months of treatment.[18] This agent has an advantage of a lower side effect profile and cost-effectiveness.

Biological agents have been effectively used in recalcitrant palmoplantar psoriasis. In a randomized controlled trial of 24 patients, they were randomized to receive infliximab 5 mg/kg or placebo at weeks 0, 2 and 6. Significant improvement of disease was seen with infliximab after 14 weeks, with no significant adverse effects.[35] Twenty subjects with moderate-to-severe psoriasis of the palms and soles were treated with ustekinumab at weeks 0, 4, and 16, in an open label trial, with a dose of 45 mg subcutaneously per week for subjects weighing <100 kg and 90 mg for those >100 kg. After 16 weeks of treatment, 35% patients achieved clinical clearance. On further analysis, it was found that 67% of those receiving the 90 mg ustekinumab dose achieved clinical clearance compared to only 9% receiving 45 mg. Thus, it was concluded that ustekinumab dosed at 90 mg is effective in controlling signs and symptoms of palmoplantar psoriasis.[36] Efalizumab, an anti-CD11a monoclonal antibody was used in the management of five patients with moderate to severe palmoplantar psoriasis. Significant improvement was seen in all patients, with no noticeable side effects. The mean m-PPPASI score at week 24 reduced by 86% from baseline and mean 99.3% improvement was seen in DLQI.[10] Other biological drugs which have shown efficacy in resistant cases of palmoplantar psoriasis include alefacept, adalimumab and etanercept.[37–39]

Palmoplantar psoriasis is a chronic, remitting and relapsing condition producing significant functional and social disability. It may be the sole manifestation of psoriasis or occurs in association with the other morphological variants. Nail changes of psoriasis are observed in 20–40% cases and arthritis may occur in 5–10% cases. Close differential diagnoses include hyperkeratotic dermatitis, pityriasis rubra pilaris, Reiter's disease, erythrokeratodermia and lichen planus. Histopathology often shows overlapping features with these conditions, therefore a clinico-pathological correlation is required.

PPP is a difficult condition to treat. Topical corticosteroids, alone or in combination with calcipotriol, coal tar, topical PUVA/PUVAsol and topical retinoids have been used with variable results. Systemic retinoids, oral PUVA, methotrexate, cyclosporine and colchicine are important systemic agents for the management of severe cases. Biological agents like ustekinumab, efalizumab, alefacept, adalimumab and etanercept have also been reported to be efficacious in recalcitrant cases.

REFERENCES

1. Pettey AA, Balkrishnan R, Rapp SR, et al. Patients with palmoplantar psoriasis have more physical disability and discomfort than patients with other forms of psoriasis: implications for clinical practice. J Am Acad Dermatol 2003;49:271–5.

2. Kumar B, Saraswat A, Kaur I. Palmoplantar lesions in psoriasis: a study of 3065 patients. Acta Derm Venereol 2002;82:192–5.

3. Venkatesan A, Aravamudhan R, Perumal SK, et al. Palmoplantar psoriasis—ahead in the race—a prospective study from a tertiary health care centre in South India. J Clin Diagn Res 2015;9:WC01–3.

4. Guinot C, Latreille J, Perrussel M, et al. Psoriasis:characterization of six different clinical phenotypes. Exp Dermatol 2009;18:712–9.

5. Khandpur S, Singhal V, Sharma VK. Palmoplantar involvement in psoriasis: a clinical study. Indian J Dermatol Venereol Leprol 2011;77:625.

6. Leibovici V, Lemster N, Ramot Y, et al. Prevalence of interdigital psoriasis of the feet ("psoriasis alba") in mild, moderate, and severe psoriasis. Int J Dermatol 2015;54:1084–7.

7. Rai R, Saraswat A, Kaur I, et al. Marginal keratoderma and psoriasis: is there an association? Int J Dermatol 2000;39:936–9.

8. Chopra A, Maninder, Gill SS. Hyperkeratosis of palms and soles: Clinical study. Indian J Dermatol Venereol Leprol 1997;63;85–8.

9. Ferrandiz C, Pujol RM, Garcia-Patos V, et al. Psoriasis of early and late onset: A clinical and epidemiologic study from Spain. J Am Acad Dermatol 2002;46:867–73.

10. Brunasso AM, Salvini C, Massone C. Efalizumab for severe palmoplantar psoriasis: an open-label pilot trial in five patients. J Eur Acad Dermatol Venereol 2009;23:415 9.

11. Aydin O, Engin B, Oguz O, et al. Non-pustular palmoplantar psoriasis: is histologic differentiation from eczematous dermatitis possible? J Cutan Pathol 2008;35:169 73.

12. Kamyab Hesari K, Naraghi ZS, Nikoo A, et al. Palmoplantar Psoriasis versus Eczema: Major Histopathologic Clues for Diagnosis. Iran J Pathol 2014:9:251–6.

13. Cesinaro AM, Nannini N, Migaldi M, et al. Psoriasis versus allergic contact dermatitis in palms and soles: a quantitative histologic and immunohistochemical study. APMIS 2009;117:629–34.

14. Quaranta M, Knapp B, Garzorz N, et al. Intra-individual genome expression analysis reveals a specific molecular signature of psoriasis and eczema. Sci Transl Med 2014;6:244ra90.

15. Garzorz N, Eyerich K. NOS2 and CCL27: clinical implications for psoriasis and eczema diagnosis and management. Expert Rev Clin Immunol 2015;11:167–9.

16. Carlén L, Sakuraba K, Ståhle M, et al. HLA-C expression pattern is spatially different between psoriasis and eczema skin lesions. J Invest Dermatol 2007;127:342–8.

17. Devillers C, Piérard-Franchimont C, Lesuisse M, et al. Overview of acquired palmoplantar keratodermas. Rev Med Liege 2011;66:535–9.

18. Adisen E, Tekin O, Gulekon A, et al. A retrospective analysis of treatment responses of palmoplantar psoriasis in 114 patients. J Eur Acad Dermatol Venereol 2009;23:814–9.

19. Kumar B, Kumar R, Kaur I. Coal tar therapy in palmoplantar psoriasis: old wine in an old bottle? Int J Dermatol 1997;36:309–12.

20. Duweb GA, Abuzariba O, Rahim M, et al. Occlusive versus non-occlusive calcipotriol ointment treatment for palmoplantar psoriasis. Int J Tissue React 2001;23:59–62.

21. Mehta BH, Amladi ST. Evaluation of topical 0.1% tazarotene cream in the treatment of palmoplantar psoriasis: an observer-blinded randomized controlled study. Indian J Dermatol 2011;56:40–3.

22. Khandpur S, Sharma VK. Comparison of clobetasol propionate cream plus coal tar vs. topical psoralen and solar ultraviolet A therapy in palmoplantar psoriasis. Clin Exp Dermatol 2011;36:613–6.

23. Kaur I, Ravi Kumar BC, Kumar B. PUVAsol therapy in palmoplantar psoriasis. Acta Derm Venereol 1996;76:491.

24. Taylor CR, Baron ED. Hand and foot PUVA soaks: an audit of the Massachusetts General Hospital's experience from 1994 to 1998. Photodermatol Photoimmunol Photomed 1999;15:188–92.

25. Carrascosa JM, Plana A, Ferrándiz C. Effectiveness and safety of psoralen-UVA (PUVA) topical therapy in palmoplantar psoriasis: a report on 48 patients. Actas Dermosifiliogr 2013;104:418–25.

26. Neumann NJ, Mahnke N, Korpusik D, et al. Treatment of palmoplantar psoriasis with monochromatic excimer light (308 nm) versus cream PUVA. Acta Derm Venereol 2006;86:22–4.

27. Hofer A, Fink-Puches R, Kerl H, et al. Paired comparison of bathwater versus oral delivery of 8-methoxypsoralen in psoralen plus ultraviolet: a therapy for chronic palmoplantar psoriasis. Photodermatol Photoimmunol Photomed 2006;22:1–5.

28. Sezer E, Erbil AH, Kurumlu Z, et al. Comparison of the efficacy of local narrowband ultraviolet B (NB-UVB) phototherapy versus psoralen plus ultraviolet A (PUVA) paint for palmoplantar psoriasis. J Dermatol 2007;34:435–40.

29. Spuls PI, Hadi S, Rivera L, et al. Retrospective analysis of the treatment of psoriasis of the palms and soles. J Dermatolog Treat 2003;14:21–5.

30. Janagond AB, Kanwar AJ, Handa S. Efficacy and safety of systemic methotrexate vs acitretin in psoriasis patients with significant palmoplantar involvement: a prospective, randomized study. J Eur Acad Dermatol Venereol 2013;27:e384–9.

31. Kumar B, Sandhu K, Kaur I. Topical 0.25% methotrexate gel in a hydrogel base for palmoplantar psoriasis. J Dermatol 2004;31:798–801.

32. Peter RU, Färber L, Weiâ J, et al. Low-dose cyclosporin A in palmoplantar psoriasis: evaluation of efficacy and safety. J Eur Acad Dermatol Venereol 1994:3:518–24.

33. Thestrup-Pedersen K, Reymann F. Treatment of Pustulosis palmaris etplantaris with colchicine. Acta Derm Venereol 1984;64:76–8.

34. Wong SS, Tan KC, Goh CL. Long-term colchicine for recalcitrant palmoplantar pustulosis: treatment outcome in 3 patients. Cutis 2001; 68:216–8.

35. Bissonnette R, Poulin Y, Guenther L, et al. Treatment of palmoplantar psoriasis with infliximab: a randomized, double-blind placebo-controlled study. J Eur Acad Dermatol Venereol 2011;25:1402–8.

36. Au SC, Goldminz AM, Kim N, et al. Investigator-initiated, open-label trial of ustekinumab for the treatment of moderate-to-severe palmoplantar psoriasis. J Dermatolog Treat 2013;24:179–87.

37. Lior S, Grigory K, Pnina S, et al. Therapeutic hotline. Alefacept in the treatment of hyperkeratotic palmoplantar psoriasis. Dermatol Ther 2010; 23:556–60.

38. Ghate JV, Alspaugh CD. Adalimumab in the management of palmoplantar psoriasis. J Drugs Dermatol 2009:8:1136–9.

39. Weinberg JM. Successful treatment of recalcitrant palmoplantar psoriasis with etanercept. Cutis 2003:72:396–8.

Index